away with

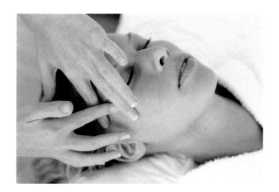

wrinkles

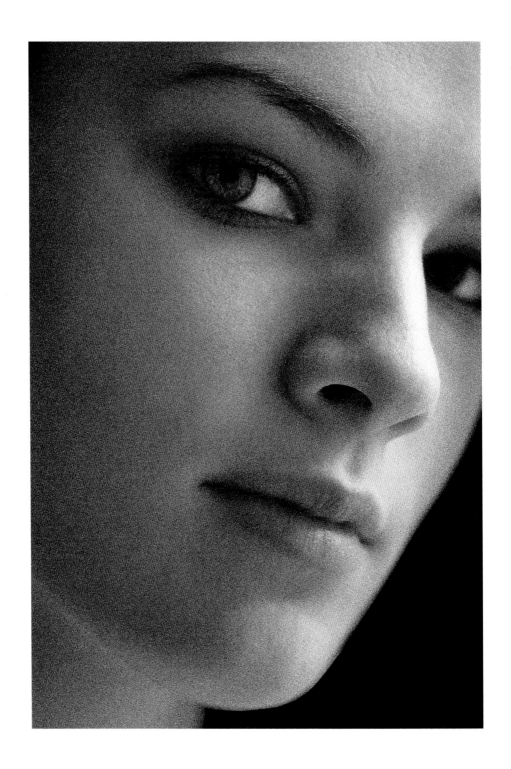

away with wrinkles

A top dermatologist's secrets for a younger face

Dr Nick Lowe

Kyle Cathie Limited

First published in Great Britain in 2005 by
Kyle Cathie Limited
122 Arlington Road
London NW1 7HP
general.enquiries@kyle-cathie.com
www.kylecathie.com

10 9 8 7 6 5 4 3 2 1

ISBN 1 85626 590 0

Nicholas Lowe is hereby identified as the author of this work in accordance with
Section 77 of the Copyright, Designs and Patents Act 1988.

Text © 2005 Nicholas Lowe
Photography © see acknowledgements on page 157
Book design © 2005 Kyle Cathie Limited

Senior Editor: Muna Reyal
Designer: Robert Updegraff
Copy editor: Anne Newman
Picture research: Jennifer Wheatley
Production: Sha Huxtable and Alice Holloway

A Cataloguing In Publication record for this title is available from the
British Library.

Colour reproduction by Scanhouse
Printed in China

contents

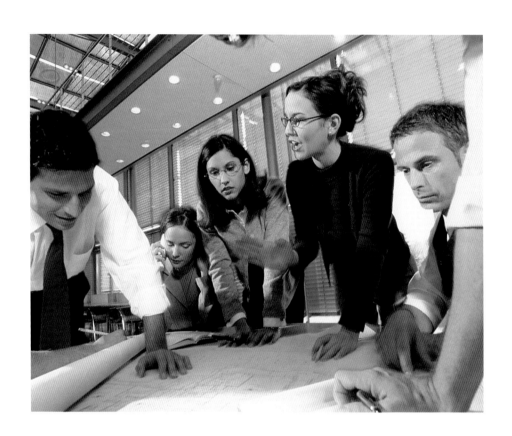

introduction

While facial ageing is an inevitable outward sign of the ageing process as a whole, this does not mean that we should not want to delay or prevent it as far as possible. People in the developed world are living longer now than ever before and treatments that allow us to look as youthful and as attractive as possible are, consequently, more in demand. After all, they are able to give us something that can offer social, personal and professional advantages.

Whether we like it or not physical attractiveness does appear to confer some advantages in life. Good-looking people are often treated better by society. They might be indulged and more easily forgiven, as Nancy Etcoff writes in *Survival of the Prettiest: the Science of Beauty*: 'Good-looking adults are more likely to get away with anything from shoplifting to cheating at exams.'

So why have I written this book? Walking through Kensington Gardens in London on a beautiful autumnal morning, I reflected on this question. The leaves had started to change colour and fall off their trees, and yet the park still remained attractive, not least through the dedicated work of the park's gardeners, tidying, trimming and pruning. This led me to think of our gradual facial ageing process and how, like autumn, its appearance can be enhanced by both Nature and man. With facial ageing, the skills of the best skin-care practitioners and their palette of rejuvenating treatments may be likened to the work of the gardeners, both resulting in the best possible appearance.

I wanted the book to be a guide for people through an area that can be confusing and quite daunting to the uninitiated: that of the many skin rejuvenation treatments now available, what they can and cannot achieve, how they work, and what to expect before, during and after.

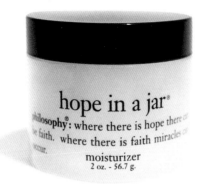

Nowadays, creams and lotions can help to protect and renew skin, but choose wisely – the best are not necessarily the most expensive.

Another reason was to explode some of the myths that surround many treatments, as all too often anti-ageing claims are based on little or no scientific evidence. With so much advertising and media hype clamouring for the public's attention it can often be difficult to separate the truth from the half-truths or even lies. These are issues that are addressed throughout the book.

Concern regarding many of the skin-care 'professionals' currently in practice was another motivation for writing this book. While the specific details and emphasis of a dermatologist's or a plastic surgeon's training might vary from country to country, *all* dermatology physicians and surgeons should undergo rigorous training in their speciality within the framework of a recognised training programme. This will mean that they will be assessed in all aspects of their speciality by medical examining boards or speciality colleges.

All too often, however, non-specialist physicians, surgeons and non-physicians claim to be specialists in the skin and cosmetic procedures, yet are not trained or qualified to carry out many of the procedures described in this book. The result, of course, is inferior standards of care, poor results and often complications. I have therefore tried to help readers to negotiate this potential minefield with sound advice on finding suitably qualified practitioners (see the Appendix, pages 144–153).

The skin is the largest organ in the body. It acts as a mirror for much of what is going on inside the body, reflecting good or bad health, and as such can be a very useful diagnostic tool. Chapter 1, therefore, looks at the skin's structure and functions and how sunlight and other factors can cause skin ageing. Chapter 2 discusses different skin types and individual signs and symptoms of ageing. This goes hand-in-hand with chapter 3 – an in-depth look at the various treatment options available, from lasers and liposuction to chemical peels and Botox injections.

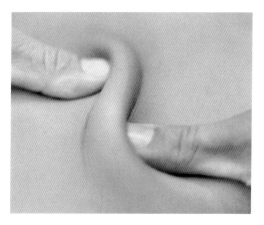

Healthy skin has amazing resilience and elasticity which allows lots of movement as well as the ability to spring back into place.

Chapter 4 is a journey through the world of cosmetic creams, cosmeceuticals, serums and sunscreens – which ones live up to their claims and which do not? And is a more expensive product always a better one? General lifestyle habits and choices and how these impact on our skin are discussed in chapter 5, as well as advice and suggestions for daily skin-care routines. Finally, in chapter 6 I look through my crystal ball to predict the future of skin rejuvenation.

I hope that having read *Away With Wrinkles* you will feel informed, inspired and empowered to make the choices that are right for you.

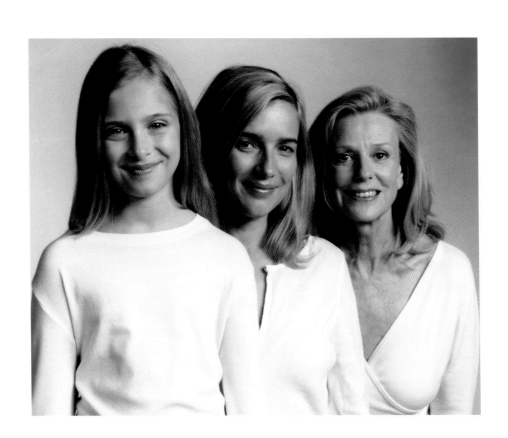

chapter one

why and how does the face age?

Facial ageing is an inevitable outward sign of the ageing process in general. Having said that, however, it can be accelerated significantly by certain habits and, conversely, delayed by positive lifestyle changes and some treatments. These need not impinge on your enjoyment of life and may well be beneficial for your health and well-being as a whole. A simple example is smoking: quitting is not only advantageous to your overall health, it is also helpful in slowing the rate at which your skin ages.

However, before we can really appreciate the whys and wherefores of facial ageing and how best to tackle it, we need to understand more fully just what the skin is and also what it does.

about your skin

The skin is the largest organ of the body and as such it is vital in maintaining general health. For example, if a person sustains burns affecting 50 per cent or more of their skin area, their health may be severely compromised and they may even be at risk of dying. Of course, our skin is also in a sense our ambassador to the outside world. We are often judged (rightly or wrongly) according to the appearance of our skin and how healthy and attractive it makes us seem to people around us. Most people are therefore conscious of how their skin looks, and try to keep it looking clear, smooth, healthy and glowing. A few people are lucky enough to have skin that looks this way naturally, but the majority of us need to learn how to treat our skin in order to achieve this goal.

skin structure

The skin is essentially made up of three different layers: the outermost layer, or epidermis; the middle supporting layer, known as the dermis; and the lowest or subcutaneous layer (see illustration below).

The epidermis

The epidermis is itself divided into several layers. The most frequently occurring epidermal cell is called the keratinocyte, or cornifying cells. These are produced in the lower levels of the epidermis and then migrate gradually outwards over a two-week period. The outermost part of the epidermis is known as the stratum corneum or horny layer and by the time the keratinocytes reach this part of the epidermis they have changed from plump round cells with nuclei to flattened cells that have started to lose their nucleus. This takes another two weeks. This process is known as cornification and is important in helping the skin to fulfil its function as a barrier. The epidermis can be thought of as the icing on top of a cake. It is thickest on the palms and soles and thinnest on the eyelids.

The dermis

This may be thought of as the marzipan layer of a cake. It is thicker than the icing (the epidermis), particularly, for example, on the scalp where it has to support hair growth. The dermis is composed of about 95 per cent collagen and 5 per cent elastin. These form the skin's supporting structure and help it to act as a shock absorber. Although there is only 5 per cent elastin, or elastic tissue, it is very efficient in helping the skin to spring back when necessary. The dermis also helps to maintain the supply of nutrients,

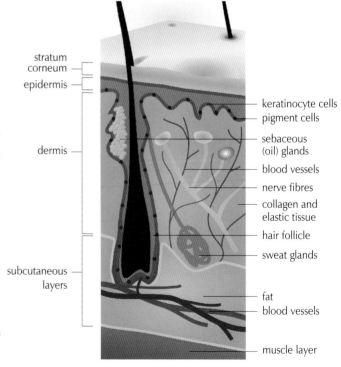

stratum corneum
epidermis
dermis
subcutaneous layers

keratinocyte cells
pigment cells
sebaceous (oil) glands
blood vessels
nerve fibres
collagen and elastic tissue
hair follicle
sweat glands
fat
blood vessels
muscle layer

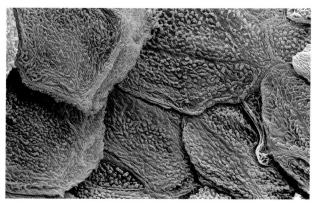

The skin's surface under an electronmicroscope – see how the cells overlap and protect your skin.

water and electrolytes to the epidermis which are essential for normal function. The dermis is thickest on places like the scalp and back, and thinnest on the eyelids.

The subcutaneous layer

If the epidermis is the icing on the cake, and the dermis the marzipan, then the subcutaneous layer would have to be the substance of the cake itself. It consists mainly of fat, crisscrossed by blood vessels, nerve fibres and fibrous cells. Its thickness varies so that it can be centimetres thick over the buttocks but very thin indeed on the eyelids, for example. It is vital in the maintenance of normal skin function and can also contribute significantly to skin ageing through the migration and loss of subcutaneous fat from various parts of the skin. Most commonly this loss of fat occurs in the face and cheeks, whereas (particularly in women) the fat lasts longest in the thighs, buttocks and abdomen. This is probably a feature related to the need for 'emergency' fat supplies in times of famine or starvation – women are much better survivors than most men!

* **How large is your skin?** *

We know that the skin is the largest organ in the body, but just how big is it? In the average adult the skin measures 2 square metres (2$\frac{1}{2}$ square yards) in area. The epidermis plus dermis are at their thickest on the soles of the feet (around 4mm ($\frac{1}{8}$in) thick) and palms of the hand and at their thinnest, in most people, on the eyelids. They weigh, on average, a total of about 4kg (9lb) and make up about 7 per cent of your total body weight.

- It protects the internal systems of your body and acts as a barrier against harmful external factors such as infections, chemicals, ultraviolet light and sunlight.

- It helps to keep water, electrolytes and other vital substances where they belong within your body.

- It helps to regulate your body temperature through sweating and controls heat loss through its blood vessels – if you are hot the blood vessels enlarge, thereby losing more heat; if you are cold they contract to conserve body heat.

- It acts as your sensation point to your environment, allowing you to feel pain, for example, as a warning that you are about to be harmed.

- It plays an important role in your appearance and therefore in the way in which you communicate with those around you and how they perceive you.

the dermatological detective

Unlike your internal organs, the skin is obviously on permanent display, which gives it some useful benefits. By learning to examine and selectively analyse a person's skin it is possible for the dermatologist to make diagnoses that can be very important to their internal health.

One example of this is highlighting internal diseases such as lupus erythematosus (a sunlight sensitivity disease) that also affects joints (arthritis) lungs as well as skin. Another example is inflammation of the blood vessels, which is known as vasculitis. Some types of vasculitis show typical patterns in the skin that can help in forming a diagnosis of the underlying disease. Some internal cancers can show up in the skin, as a change in skin colour, for example, whereas other types may spread to the skin and show as smooth lumps. Liver disease can be manifested in the skin as extensive spider veins, a redness of the palms and sometimes a yellow complexion.

pigmentation

The epidermis (see page 12) is home to the pigment cells, also known as melanocytes, which produce pigment or melanin. The melanocyte is the factory in which a suntan is manufactured.

Unfortunately, people with red hair have a relatively inefficient type of melanin called phaeomelanin. This protects very poorly against sunlight making them prone to skin cancers and accelerated skin ageing. Other types of skin that tan more efficiently, such as phototypes 2–6 (see pages 28–29), produce a type of melanin called eumelanin. This is much more efficient at repairing the damage caused by sunlight and also at producing a protective tan.

It is through an intriguing mechanism called pigment transfer that a tan is distributed from the melanocytes to all the keratinocytes (see page 12). There is good evidence that black skin is much more efficient at this melanin transfer. This is because although all skin types have the same ratio (1:10) of melanocytes to keratinocytes, the darker the skin the more efficient the melanin that is produced and therefore the more efficient the pigment transfer. (See also page 29.) The epidermis also thickens in response to sunlight, therefore affording more protection from subsequent sunlight exposure.

causes of skin ageing

Now let's take a look at the main causes of skin ageing.

Photoageing

The main reason for premature ageing of the skin is sun damage, or photoageing. In fact, over 90 per cent of the therapies used for rejuvenation are aimed at damage that has occurred as a direct result of repeated exposure to sunlight.

Skin and facial ageing is caused by the following factors:

- Photoageing – caused by repeated exposure to sunlight
- Smoking
- Alcohol
- Diet
- Increased activity of some facial muscles
- Loss of fat from cheeks
- Movement of fat to jowls and lower eyelids (fat pads)

Sunlight is made up of different wavelengths of light. The earth's atmosphere shields us from x-rays, but allows visible light, ultraviolet A (UVA) and ultraviolet B (UVB) through. This light causes the skin to age before it should – i.e. prematurely – by directly breaking down its supporting structures, collagen and elastin. It also damages the enzymes that protect collagen from breakdown. UVB mainly increases skin cancer while UVA mainly increases skin ageing.

The UVA part of sunlight, comprising longer wavelengths, can penetrate through to the deeper skin, and there has also been important research

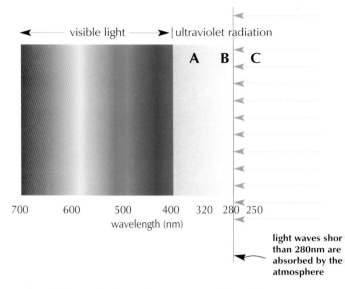

The visible and ultraviolet portions of the solar spectrum. The UV portion is normally divided into three segments: A is the long-wave portion and causes skin cancer and skin ageing; B is known as the erythemogenic portion and causes sunburn and skin cancer; and C is the short-wave portion and does not usually reach the earth's surface because the short wavelengths are absorbed by the atmosphere. This may change with ozone depletion and at high altitude.

pointing to the fact that it can even pass through glass. This means that simply by sitting in your car in daylight hours without applying sunscreen you will cause the skin to age because the car windows do not contain ultraviolet filters. If you drive on the left side of the road and take a look at your right hand you may well notice a subtle or definite increase in ageing when compared with the left hand. Equally, some people in the UK notice that the right side of their face ages more quickly than the left, again because of driving on the left. In other countries around the world, the USA for example, the reverse can be seen and drivers experience increased sun damage on the left side of the face and the left hand and arm.

How is sunlight damage manifested?

- Surface damage results in red or brown blemishes and more prominent blood vessels (thread veins or spider veins, see page 30).

- Fine wrinkles and sallowness of the skin can be caused by damage to the under carpet of the skin (the dermis) and to the collagen and elastic tissue. These are damaged both directly by the sun itself and by sunburn which produces inflammation leading to the breakdown of collagen and elastic fibres.

- Causes pre-skin cancer (solar keratoses, see page 31) and skin cancers.

This is something I see very clearly when comparing a fair-skinned person who has lived in the UK with their southern Californian counterpart – generally the Californian's skin will look a good five to ten years older (unless the British person is a sun or tanning-bed addict). The effects of more intense sunlight in California are compounded by the fact that sunscreen ingredients in the USA are not as effective as those in the UK (see chapter 4).

Tanning machines

These are, in my opinion, second only to smoking as a significant public health concern. People persist in using tanning machines in the mistaken belief that a tanned skin is a healthy one, when it is actually a sign of injury, causing accelerated ageing of the skin. Tanning machines produce huge quantities of long-wave ultraviolet (UVA). This was believed to be much safer than the sunburn spectrum (UVB); however, it is now known that these can reach much deeper, leading to sagging and wrinkling, and also to an increased risk of some skin cancers, including potentially fatal melanomas.

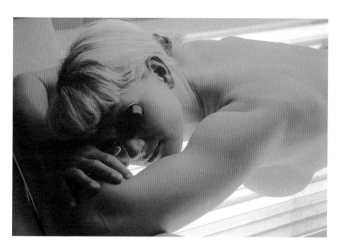

Tanning machines are very dangerous to the skin and should not be seen as a safe alternative to sunbathing.

Unfortunately, while there are recommendations for tanning machine operators to follow (regarding people on certain medications and pregnant women and so on), there is no formal legal obligation and a recent survey suggested that these recommendations were not complied with.

Other complications that can arise from the use of tanning machines include:

- skin darkening during pregnancy in women who are prone to facial pigmentation

- a severe sunburn reaction known as phototoxicity in people on medications such as antibiotics, oral contraceptives, water tablets and some anti-diabetes tablets, resulting in blistering and burning.

Other weather conditions

It is not only sunlight that can affect the skin. Wind, rain, cold, heat and sudden changes in temperature can all take their toll. Exposure to water can break down the skin barrier and increase dryness as a result; changes from hot to cold or cold to hot can cause a rapid increase in the size of blood vessels leading to a 'weather-beaten' appearance and a very ruddy complexion. People who either work outdoors or who do a lot of outdoor sports or activities without adequate sun protection are prone to these problems.

Smoking

Smoking has been shown to cause skin ageing for several reasons.

Firstly, it reduces the amount of oxygen supply to all body organs including the skin by narrowing the blood vessels. This in turn causes the skin to function much less efficiently and that means that less collagen and elastin are produced. Smokers' blood does not carry as much oxygen as that of non-smokers.

Smoking also causes premature skin ageing because it damages one of the enzymes which controls the production of collagen in the skin. I recently saw a woman in her mid-40s whom I persuaded to give up smoking and take regular exercise. The result, some four months later, was remarkable: she not only looked at least ten years younger, she also felt much better about herself.

Alcohol

Alcohol is a factor in certain types of skin ageing. It can cause repeated then constant enlargement of the blood vessels resulting in the characteristic red-faced appearance of many drinkers. Repeated reddening leads to spider veins. Excess alcohol can also reduce the absorption of key vitamins and the nutrients that the skin requires.

Diet

Rapid and severe dietary restrictions geared towards weight loss can cause skin sagging on the face, as well as other parts of the body (such as breasts, stomach, arms and thighs). As the skin ages it becomes less efficient at compensating for rapid changes in the amount of supporting fat under the skin. Sagging therefore occurs, leading to a markedly older appearance. Gradual, steady weight loss is much more beneficial from the point of view of general health, for a longer and more active life, and, of course, a better-looking skin.

Stretch marks can be another by-product of gaining and losing weight rapidly (their most common cause is pregnancy). They are essentially a widening or stretching of the collagen and elastin bundles and can vary in colour. Fresh stretch marks are a pinkish colour, but as they age they become more silvery in appearance. Possible treatments for stretch marks include the use of topical Retin-A type creams, microdermabrasion and some laser treatments (see pages 107, 56 and 58).

Drug and substance abuse, as well as causing internal health problems in themselves, can also lead to poor dietary habits and sudden weight loss. All these together with smoking and sun exposure combine to age the skin much more than is necessary.

Increased activity of some facial muscles

There is a myth created by some writers and 'beauty experts' that good muscle tone is essential if the face is to remain youthful-looking. This is likely to be true in some areas such as the lower face, the cheeks and possibly the neck. However, in some people increased muscle activity in, for example, the forehead, around the eyes and around the mouth, can lead to an increase in the number of lines. These can, however, be reduced with treatments such as the use of botulinum toxin (Botox, see chapter 3).

* Genetic factors *

Genetic predisposition plays a big part in the way in which your skin ages. The question is what can be done about it? Clearly we cannot (at the moment, at least) reverse the genes we are given. What may be important, however, is to observe how your parents have aged and see if there are any lifestyle factors (smoking, excessive sun exposure, dietary habits, for example) that might have led to increased facial and skin ageing. The likelihood is that if they have caused ageing in your parents, there is a good chance that they will interact with genetic factors in you to create the same effect.

what can be done to reduce the skin-ageing problem?

There are many treatments available and these will be discussed during the course of this book. However, *it is never too early or too late* to start thinking about skin protection, skin renewal and maintenance treatment.

As the populations of northern Europe, northern USA and Canada have become more affluent, there has been a corresponding increase in travel to sunny climates and, therefore, in sun exposure. Awareness and use of *effective* sunscreens (and by no means all are effective, see page 114) are therefore essential as these will protect while your skin repairs.

The important thing to remember is that protecting and enjoying yourself outdoors need not be mutually exclusive. The vast majority of people are able to protect themselves with effective sunscreens and sun-protective clothing, and in so doing they enjoy a normal healthy outdoor lifestyle while minimising any damage from the sun. Only a small percentage of the population suffer from sun sensitivity diseases which means that they do have to greatly restrict their activities.

It is vital to keep to a regime in which you protect yourself every morning with sunscreen to reduce the causes of accelerated skin ageing and apply nourishing and repair creams at night (see Skin-care Routines, page 130). In this way the two do not interfere with each other. Individual sunscreens and creams will be discussed in more detail later in the book (see pages 112–113).

When should you start thinking about starting sun protection, skin renewal and maintenance?

Many of the teenagers and pre-teens I come across seem to believe they are invincible and that they do not need to follow any sort of skin protection programme. However, as I said earlier, it is never too early to start. Parents should make a point of educating and training their children in taking sun protection measures as well as general healthy lifestyle habits. Schools and the public health services, as well as bodies like the British Association of Dermatologists, the Skin Care Campaign in the UK, the American Academy of Dermatology and several cancer organisations also have a very important role to play in public education.

What can you do yourself?

- Use a sunscreen in sunny weather in northern Europe or the north-eastern United States from the middle of spring to the middle of autumn (see pages 112–114 for recommendations on sunscreens). If you are prone to skin cancer, to dark skin areas or you already have sun damage you should use a sunscreen all year round.

- If you go skiing in the winter remember to use a good 'broad-spectrum' sunscreen (see page 112) plus a hat, ski mask and UV-protecting sunglasses. High altitude means thinner atmosphere and therefore greater UV exposure.

- If you are in your 20s and you start to notice the early signs of sun damage (particularly early wrinkling, some darker sunspots ('age' spots) or masks of pigmentation from pregnancy or the pill) you should consult a dermatologist and discuss with them the use of sun-protection programmes, prescriptive skin-lightening creams (unfortunately the strength of most of the non-prescription skin-lightening creams is not particularly effective), and other treatments that I can recommend such as lasers and chemical peels (see chapter 3).

> ## Always remember ...
>
> - A suntanned skin is a *damaged* skin. Use sunless self-tanning solutions if you want a tanned look (see pages 114–115).
>
> - Expensive creams that contain sunscreens may not provide adequate protection against sunlight-accelerated skin ageing. See my recommendations for sunscreens in chapter 4.

- If you drink alcohol and notice that you are readily flushing, try reducing or cutting out alcohol or switching to an alternative type of alcoholic drink that may reduce this problem.

- Try to eat a sensible, steady diet. Avoid sudden weight gain and crash dieting (see above) and take appropriate vitamin supplements (see page 128).

- Use good skin treatment and maintenance creams. These will be discussed in detail in chapter 4, but it is important to note here that many cosmetic and so-called 'cosmeceutical' creams make false and misleading claims, exaggerating their benefits and effects on the skin. The skin can repair itself to a degree and this process can be significantly enhanced with the use of appropriate protection and treatment creams; however, it is vital to ensure that there is strong scientific evidence to back up their claims (see chapter 4).

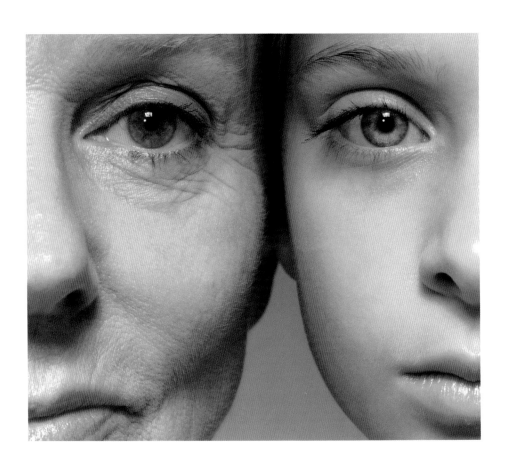

chapter two

problems and solutions

Each and every one of us is unique, and it follows, therefore, that every one of us is different as regards our skin type and the way in which our skin ages. Ageing is governed by a number of factors, as discussed in the previous chapter, but the process itself is manifested in various ways. In this chapter, we will be looking at all the various signs of ageing, along with some suggestions on how best to tackle them.

when and how do people age?

As I have already mentioned, each of us is different and your particular signs of ageing will be governed largely by factors such as how well your skin has been protected and the climate in which you live as well as lifestyle habits such as smoking. However, it is possible to draw up a rough guide to demonstrate when the average person can expect to see the first signs of facial ageing, and what these might be.

* Beware! *

As a general rule, the more you are exposed to sunlight with inadequate protection, and particularly if you have smoked, the younger you will be when the first signs of facial ageing start to creep in!

Teenage years

In your teenage years, your skin should look bright and clear unless you have problems with acne. In most teenagers this is caused by normal hormone changes, which, these days, can start even before the teenage years with many young people maturing earlier. The hormones, which are called androgens, increase the production of the oil sebum that is produced by the oil or sebaceous glands. The sebum flows from the sebaceous glands and the hormones also act to block the opening of the oil ducts, thus producing blackheads and whiteheads. The blackhead is a blockage that is open to the air and has become black. A whitehead is a blockage that is not open to the air and, therefore, stays white.

Behind these blocked pores, the acne bacteria grow more rapidly within the sebaceous glands and produce the inflammation and redness that characterise the condition. Treatment of acne will be dealt with later (see page 34) but suffice it to say there are many different treatments for acne and a consultant dermatologist will be able to help and advise you. (See also Appendix, page 144.)

Generally speaking, however, in your teens the cells of your skin are being produced at an optimum rate, your dermis is nice and plump and the collagen and elastin are functioning normally with good elasticity and resilience. In other words, your skin should be in peak condition apart, possibly, from some acne.

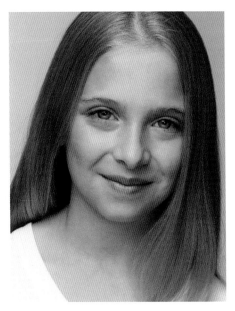

You have good, firm elastic skin with no wrinkles when your face is at rest. Lucky you – learn to keep it that way for as long as possible.

20s

When you get to your 20s, your skin should be reasonably smooth without any major lines unless you have lived in a very sunny place and been overly exposed to sunburn from an early age. Fair skin that is exposed to excessive sunlight during childhood can start to show signs of facial changes as early as the 20s (whereas the same skin that has been protected may not show any signs until 10 to 20 years later).

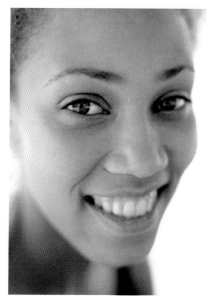

These changes may not necessarily manifest themselves so much as lines and wrinkles at this stage, but more as the beginnings of sunspots (see page 36). If you have sustained a lot of sunlight damage, towards the end of your 20s you may start to see some early lines, particularly crow's feet around the sides of your eyes.

30s

Between the ages of 30 and 40, the appearance of your skin will, again, depend largely on how well it has been protected from sunlight, although this is also the point at which genetic factors may kick in (see page 19). If your skin is starting to look dull at this stage (which it may well do, especially if you

Your skin is still smooth, blemish-free and largely unwrinkled.

are a smoker) with the appearance of more sunspots and maybe even some small, scaly, red precancerous skin lesions (see page 31), then it is worth thinking about consulting a dermatologist for one of the prescription-type cream treatments described on page 107. Another option to consider would be the use of microdermabrasion and superficial peels together with intense pulsed light (see pages 56 and 63) if wrinkles are starting to show.

One of the other problems that can occur in the 30s is creasing of the skin from repeated muscle activity. This can cause the start of a central frown line, forehead lines and more crow's feet. An ideal treatment (as well as a preventative approach) is to start using Botox injections (see pages 73–78) but these should only be carried out by a specialist dermatologist or plastic surgeon who should inject it themselves and not delegate to a staff member.

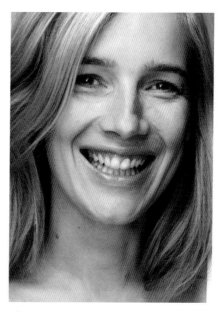

Skin treatments may help you to look even better.

40s–50s

At this stage your skin is significantly more likely to show the signs of past sun exposure, as well as increased frown and smile lines from muscle activity. Generally speaking, you should not (unless you have a strong family history) start showing a loss of fat under the skin with loss of firmness, although some plumpness in the lips may be lost and lines on the lower face may appear. Smokers will have more lines around the eyes and mouth. In addition to the other treatments listed previously including Botox, you might want to consider hyaluronic acid or NewFill fillers (see pages 79–84) for lower facial lines. Fat transfer (see page 85) can also be used successfully.

If you are developing sunspots, spider veins and thread veins, these can be treated with a laser. Laser resurfacing is an option for sun-damaged skin.

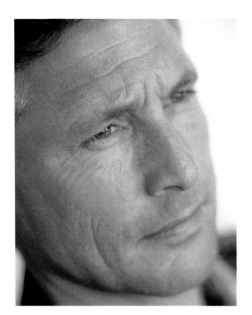

You are an ideal candidate for Botox and fillers as well as the treatment of red skin and thread veins.

50s–60s

At this stage, you will probably be experiencing a general worsening of all the above, as well as feeling a greater change under the skin with a sagging eyelid and/or brow droop. For this you may want to obtain a referral for eyelid surgery and try lower facial fillers to rejuvenate the face and cheeks. Skin lines will be more noticeable, and sunspots and precancerous spots will show. Laser resurfacing (see page 68), if you have already tried prescription rejuvenation creams, and chemical peels will be helpful.

You will see deeper facial lines and signs of sun damage with eye shadows and blotches.

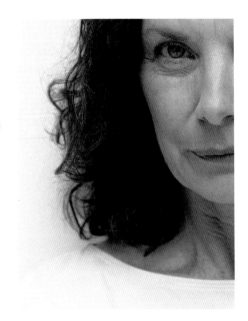

60s, 70s and beyond

From your 60s, 70s and onwards, if you have had a lot of sun exposure then your lines and brown spots will start ageing the skin more severely and it is here that UltraPulse carbon dioxide laser resurfacing can be of real benefit. It looks extremely natural and is highly effective at rejuvenating the face. As mentioned previously, it is of paramount importance to go to somebody who is trained in dermatology and in laser skin therapy. Again, for spider veins and brown spots, the use of the other appropriate lasers is very helpful.

Continued use of prescription strengths of Retin-A as well as maintenance chemical peels and sun protection are all very important, along with pulsed light rejuvenation therapy for keeping the face looking youthful.

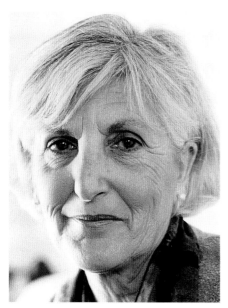

An attractive, but lined face. There are now numerous non-surgical treatments if you want to look more youthful.

To conclude

As we have seen, your skin will age according to your skin type, genetic factors and lifestyle choices. You may not want to erase all of life's imprint from your face and neck, but it is possible to do much to soften its touch.

Start thinking about skin care, especially sun protection, as early as you can. Choose well-formulated sunscreens (see chapter 4) and a good cleansing routine as well as a healthy diet (see chapter 5) and you will see the benefits for many years ahead. Ignoring these factors will mean that you will age faster.

There will come a time, however, when the signs of ageing can no longer be held at bay, but there are plenty of non-invasive, non-surgical options. Before we look at these, however, I would like to explain the six skin types and then discuss in detail the key signs of ageing and their causes.

skin types

There are six basic skin types, which are known medically by numbers and are classified on the basis of fairness (or otherwise) of skin, eye and hair colour and the skin's tendency either to burn or tan in response to exposure to sunlight. They may be summarised as follows:

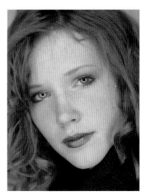

Skin Phototype 1

People with this skin type burn very easily and rarely tan. They are most likely to have very light blond hair or red hair and freckles. Red-heads have an inefficient type of melanin.

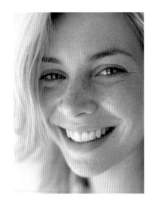
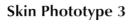

Skin Phototype 2

Skin in this range always burns but will also tan slightly. It is a fairish colour and usually goes with blue eyes, and blond or light brown hair. There may be some exceptions – some people of Celtic origin who may have extremely sun-sensitive phototype 1 or 2 skin with black hair.

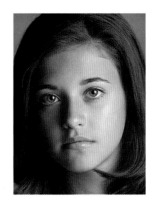

Skin Phototype 3

This type is a light olive colour, usually with brown or green eyes and dark hair. Skin will burn if overexposed but will always develop a medium to dark tan.

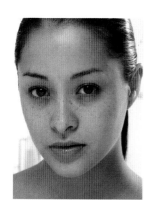

Skin Phototype 4

This skin is a darker olive in colour, usually with brown eyes and dark hair. Skin can burn slightly but always tans deeply and quickly.

Skin Phototype 5

This type is a brown to light black, usually with brown eyes and dark hair. Sunburn is minimal and the skin tans briskly and deeply.

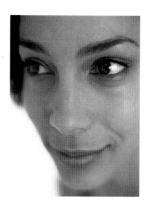

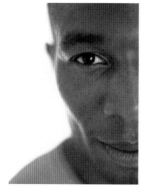

Skin Phototype 6

This is a darker black skin type with brown eyes and dark hair. The skin does not burn easily and tans very deeply.

Phototypes 2–6 have a more efficient and protective type of melanin.

(For information on how to protect different skin types from the effects of the sun, see page 113.)

How protective is a darker skin?

It is estimated that black skin offers a natural sun protection factor (SPF) of about 6, dark Asian skin 4–5 and Mediterranean olive skin about 3. The protection goes beyond that of its SPF value, however, as the melanin tan also acts as an effective free radical-quenching factory that absorbs, soaks up and repairs some of the damage caused by sunlight and other factors.

skin changes: what they are and how they are caused

While everybody has their own individual skin type which will age and wrinkle differently, there are several signs of ageing that are common to all.

Spider veins and thread veins

Lighter skin types are more prone to spider veins – enlarged blood vessels on the skin's surface that can appear as little straight red lines (thread veins), red marks, or as a central spot with a web-like red surround, like a spider's web (hence the name). They can be inherited genetically, or may result from frequent exposure to rapid changes in temperature, or to windy weather. They can also be a response to alcohol. They occur most commonly on the face, neck and chest, and while they may be distressing from a cosmetic point of view they are not, in most cases, a health concern. However, in a small minority, spider veins may be caused by an underlying problem such as liver, thyroid or other diseases that produce excess hormones. A dermatologist will be able to determine this, and advise you accordingly. The most likely course of treatment would be with a pulsed dye laser or light machine that targets enlarged blood vessels (see page 58).

Precancerous spots (solar keratoses)

Another hazard for lighter skin types is precancerous spots. These are a warning sign that the skin has, in the past, been more exposed to the sun than it should have been. They are most commonly seen on the face, neck, upper chest, back of the hands and forearms. They may be flat, red and slightly scaly or they may have thicker white scaling or sometimes a brown appearance. They are not in themselves dangerous (although they can be disfiguring and ageing), but people who have them are generally more at risk of skin cancer and should therefore be checked regularly by a dermatologist. If necessary a small skin sample may be taken to ascertain whether a precancerous spot has changed into a skin cancer and treatment, if it is required, may take the form of either prescription creams, freezing with a cold spray or removal by lasers or photodynamic treatment.

Darker skin types carry a lower risk for skin cancer and pre-skin cancers and are likely to age differently, with brown uneven spots on sun-exposed skin. They are also prone to lines and wrinkles. Also, in the event of any injury to the skin or any dermatitis (skin disease such as eczema), it is likely that the skin will heal with brown pigment or lose pigment completely. Scars may be brown or more severe scars white.

Upper facial lines

If you have very intense forehead muscles in the centre of your forehead, you will find that you develop a lot of wrinkles in your forehead. These can show up either as deep vertical lines making you look angry and cross, or horizontal lines that can often make you look aggressive. The muscles that produce the vertical lines also cause a pulling down of your eyebrows, again giving an older, meaner appearance. Some people manage to reduce their forehead and smile muscle action which can, in turn, help to develop fewer lines. Ultraviolet-protective sunglasses will also help by making you squint less. Smokers usually have deeper lines as a result of squinting through their smoke, among other reasons (see page 120).

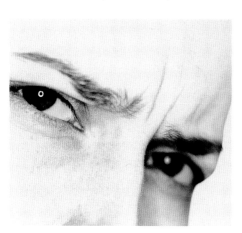

Forehead lines can make you look angry, anxious and worried.

The commonly held belief that facial muscles should be toned and exercised in order to delay ageing of the face is nothing more than a beauty-industry and media-hyped myth. In fact, for most of the face the reverse is true, and exercising the muscles of the upper face by increasing muscle action in that area can lead to a significantly increased number of lines around the eyes, the forehead and around the mouth.

It may be possible to help jaw-line and neck sagging a little with appropriate exercises.

A very effective way to deal with these upper facial lines, as well as to achieve a non-surgical browlift, is to reduce muscle action with the help of botulinum toxin which will be covered in more detail in chapter 3. Botox should only be carried out by either a trained specialist-registered dermatologist or a plastic surgeon, and not by a GP or nurse. It is a prescription medication but there are known cases in which GPs have bought it from a pharmacist and sold it on to nurses or beauty therapists. This is highly unprofessional and my advice would be to consult specialist dermatologists only.

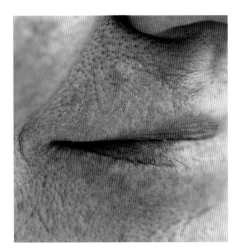

These lines are created by fat loss and facial movement.

Lower facial lines

Lower facial lines result mainly from the loss of the substance underlying your skin, i.e. the 'carpet underlay' of subcutaneous tissues beneath the skin's surface, comprising collagen, fat and muscle tissues. This occurs when some of the anchoring fat fibres become detached with age. These deeper lines are most commonly seen between the nose and the mouth, where they are known medically as nasolabial folds and also below the lips, where they are sometimes referred to as 'sad' lines.

Because lower facial lines occur largely as result of the loss of the natural support filling of the skin, the solution is to restore that support. A dermatologist or plastic surgeon will discuss with you the different fillers that can be used to plump up the lower face. These have evolved considerably in recent years and now a range of temporary short-acting, longer-acting and permanent fillers and implants is now available. Those that might be offered are likely to include Restylane-Perlane, fat transfer (your own harvested fat) and the recently developed NewFill (Sculptra). It is important to be aware that some of these treatments can cause lumps and other reactions. (For more information, see pages 83–84.) Restylane SubQ (a very recent implant) is injectable and is thought to last for several years.

Neck ageing

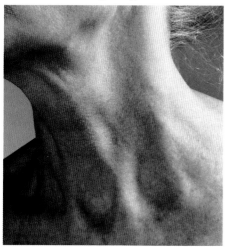

Good improvement is possible but only when done correctly.

An ageing neck can play a big part in making a person's face look older. I see many patients who have carefully protected their faces or possibly undergone some sort of facial rejuvenation and yet their necks show signs of significant sun damage.

The neck is easily damaged by sun exposure as the skin is much thinner than it is on parts of the face and its support structure is not as effective. It therefore ages more readily as a result of skin surface damage. As fat is lost from under the neck skin unsightly strands and bands of skin and muscle, often known as turkey necks, appear. Another manifestation of ageing neck skin is a double chin, which is an excessive collection of fat.

Rejuvenation treatment of the ageing neck is a very specialised area and you must ensure that your practitioner is qualified. Some of the treatments that can be used on the face may either not be used at all on the neck and chest or have to be modified for safety reasons. Some treatments to these areas can cause unpredictable problems such as scarring, skin lightening and skin redness. Treatments that are safe to use on the neck and chest include some chemical peels, photo rejuvenation and laser treatment for brown patches and red veins (see chapter 3).

＊ Sun protection for the neck ＊

Always remember that your neck and upper chest will influence how youthful you look: it is vital that you do not forget to protect and treat them with sun protection and rejuvenating creams (see pages 107–114, 118–119).

Ageing eyes

One of the most common signs of ageing eyes are crow's feet – lines around the eyes caused by repetitive smiling, sunlight ageing and smoking. Bags under the eyes can also develop due to weakness of the ligaments in the eyelids which creates a bulging of fat under the eyes. This fat is normally a natural protection for the eyeballs but in the course of ageing begins to show itself as bags, usually beneath the eyes, but sometimes above.

Drooping or extra skin in the upper eyelids is another sign of ageing eyes. This may be due to sagging of the upper lid but can also be due to sagging of the forehead skin which, in turn, leads to a drooping eyebrow.

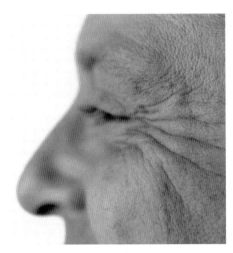

Lines caused by sun damage and smiling can be improved by combining Botox with other treatments.

The most successful treatment for crow's feet and other eye lines is a combination of rejuvenating cream such as Retin-A (see page 107), laser skin rejuvenation (see page 62), and Botox injection (see page 73). For bags around the eyes the most effective treatment is a specialised form of cosmetic surgery known as oculoplastic surgery. Laser resurfacing following surgery may be useful but would not be very successful on its own.

Skin disease

• **Acne** is a condition that occurs to a greater or lesser degree in the vast majority of people and while some only experience a few spots, others have more severe cases.

Acne usually affects the face, and sometimes the front and back of the chest, but can also appear on the lower back, buttocks and thighs. It is caused by a combination of hormonal stimuli to the acne or sebaceous glands in the skin. This in turn leads to an increased production of oil, which is accompanied by a blockage to the opening of the duct, which will be seen as a blackhead or whitehead (see also page 24). In the long term, acne also increases the breakdown of collagen and elastic tissue.

There are many new prescription treatments for acne, and older ones such as Retin-A cream which has also been proven to rejuvenate the skin. Generally speaking, acne-prone skin will tolerate treatment with peels as well as other rejuvenating treatments.

Acne: the myths and the facts

Myth Rubbing the skin too hard increases facial oil and therefore causes acne.

Fact Acne can be exacerbated (but not caused) by rubbing or friction, so the condition can often be worse in areas under visors, caps, hats or headbands.

Myth Eating chocolate causes acne.

Fact Eating chocolate does not seem to be a risk factor as such, but it may contribute to the severity of the condition although this varies from case to case.

• **Eczema** is most common in children when it is known as childhood or atopic eczema (atopic eczema is an inherited condition linked with asthma and hay fever, although neither of these conditions need be present). Around 80 per cent of children who develop eczema will have outgrown it by their teenage years. In around 20 per cent of cases, however, it can continue into adult life. Atopic eczema can also return after an absence of many years, often precipitated by triggers such as stress or irritated skin. It is important to know whether or not you are an eczema sufferer before you undergo any skin rejuvenation as some of the treatments used (alpha-hydroxy acid, Retin-A cream and chemical peels, for example) can aggravate the condition.

Allergic eczema (scaling red patches) can occur particularly on the face and may be the result of an allergy to one of the many ingredients in face lotions and creams. A dermatologist will be able to investigate this possibility further for you.

• **Psoriasis** affects around 2 per cent of the population. It manifests itself as red, scaling patches, often on the elbows and knees, but it can become more widespread. Like eczema, it is usually inherited, can remain dormant for years and then be brought out again by stress or other trigger factors.

The most important thing to know about psoriasis in terms of skin rejuvenation is that many sufferers may have already undergone ultraviolet treatment which will put them at higher risk of some skin cancers and certain skin ageing changes. Also, some procedures such as skin biopsies, laser resurfacing and some of the stronger peels can have an adverse effect on psoriasis sufferers.

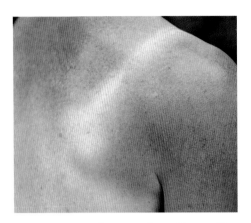

Repeated suntanning will age skin. Note the increased freckling, redness and fine lines.

Sun damage

Besides the classic burned appearance associated with too much sun exposure, other effects include uneven texture, brown and white blotches on the skin, and uneven red and brown colouring. It is mainly the 'chronically' exposed areas of skin, i.e. the face, neck, upper chest, forearms and hands that are affected.

(For more information on sun damage, sun protection and treatment options see pages 111–115, 118–119.)

Birthmarks

These can be present in a variety of shapes, sizes, colours, and locations. The most common type of birthmark is the flat, dark brown coffee-coloured spot, often referred to as a *café au lait* mark. Port-wine stains and strawberry marks are also common, usually appearing at birth or shortly afterwards. These may be treated successfully in a number of ways, most often with modern laser systems (see page 58), although many strawberry birthmarks disappear gradually on their own in time.

Rosacea

Rosacea used to be known as adult acne. It is more common in certain ethnic groups, in particular Celtic and north European people, and is characterised by flushing/blushing-like acne spots, often under the skin's surface, swelling of the nose, redness of the eyes and eyelids, and eventually spider veins (see page 30). Excellent treatments are available for rosacea including topical creams and tablets which can be prescribed by your dermatologist. Modern laser and pulsed light treatments are also highly effective. It is important to establish a diagnosis first as other diseases such as seborrhoeic eczema and lupus erythematosus can look very similar to rosacea.

Age spots

More accurately known as sunspots, they appear as flat, brown marks on the hands, face and other areas of sun-exposed skin. Treatment for these includes pigment lasers, the pulsed-light rejuvenation system (see pages 58 and 63) and prescription creams.

hair problems

Dermatologists have trained for many years to deal not only with diseases and problems of the skin but also those of the hair, so consult them about hair loss and hair and scalp disease. Your hair is of critical importance for your looks and youthfulness. In men it tends to be a symbol of virility and youthfulness, while in women it spells glamour and allure. Men and women who are balding or who have thinning hair tend to look and feel less attractive and older than their years, but new treatments can be successful.

Thinning hair

Thinning hair, which is known medically as alopecia, can either be generalised (the most common type in women and men) or localised. Hair thinning over the whole scalp, or generalised alopecia, can often stem from genetic inheritance although the genetics are not always clear cut, so that the way your parents' hair looks is not necessarily an indication of how your own will look. Sometimes you will have to look at your aunts, uncles and grandparents to find a hair-loss pattern that is similar to your own. Localised alopecia (alopecia areata) is the result of local immune damage to hair follicles for which you need to consult a dermatologist.

Other causes of thinning hair include:

- certain types of medication including some types of oral contraceptives, antidepressants, anti-cancer drugs, oral antibiotics, diabetes drugs and blood-thinning drugs

- crash weight-loss diets or diets with reduced protein, vitamin and iron intake

- underlying internal diseases such as over- and underactivity of the thyroid gland, conditions that lead to a loss of blood and iron (for example heavy periods in women, or bleeding from the bowel), some types of arthritis and rare conditions such as lupus erythematosus.

Hair loss in women

Women most commonly suffer hair loss following pregnancy and from iron and vitamin deficiency. Interestingly, hair loss can highlight an iron deficiency problem long before any blood problems such as anaemia are apparent.

It is important to ensure that your diet contains large amounts of iron and vitamins (from green vegetables and red meat, for example). Vegetarians should certainly take iron supplements. The B group of vitamins, biotin, and the daily recommended doses of vitamins A, D and E are all important to maintain good hair growth. These are marked on the packaging as RDAs (recommended daily amounts).

Women who have either recently been pregnant or who have changed or stopped the contraceptive pill may find that they experience a period of increased hair loss. This is a problem that will generally correct itself over time but sometimes the hair may not return to the density it had before. Again you need to seek the advice of a dermatologist.

Hair loss in women can be caused by surplus androgen or male hormones which can also cause acne (see page 34), as well as excess body hair growth. In such cases certain types of contraceptive pill known as Dianette and Yasmin (Spironolactone in the USA, as Dianette is not available) may be prescribed to correct the imbalance.

Stress is another factor in hair loss in women. It is important for both the dermatologist and the patient to recognise this as a possible culprit so that necessary measures can be taken such as stress relaxation, guided imagery, hypnotherapy or medication.

Tackling the Problem of Balding

A small number of women, and much larger numbers of men, experience what is known as pattern or male-pattern hair loss; the hair is lost usually from the front and upper part of the scalp and temple areas more than elsewhere. While this is quite normal in men (as the name would suggest), in women it is a problem for which advice from a dermatologist should be sought in order to rule out the possibility of disease. Other common causes include post-

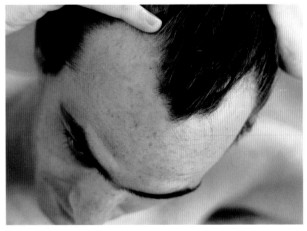

Modern treatments can really improve thinning hair, but beware of promised miracles.

pregnancy, after stopping taking an oral contraceptive pill or it may be part of generalised hair loss. More rarely, it may be due to conditions where there are excess male hormones.

The following treatments can be helpful:

- Minoxidil lotion up to 5 per cent for men and up to 2 per cent for women (known as Regaine in Europe and Rogaine in the USA). This can be bought over the counter but you should check with your dermatologist before treating yourself. Used nightly or twice daily it may be expected to increase the amount of hair growth if used over at least a six-month period and then as a maintenance treatment thereafter. It does seem to be most effective on the crown of the scalp and less so on the frontal and temple areas. It can also cause some scalp irritation and if this is the case it should be used less frequently. Interestingly, if hair loss occurs as a result of pregnancy or certain medications Rogaine/Regaine lotion, used over several months, can restore hair density which then can be long lasting.

- Prescription drugs can be used to block the effects of the male hormones that are the cause of hair loss in some women and most men. The drug that has been approved for treatment is called Propecia. It is important to be seen by your dermatologist, however, to assess whether or not you are a candidate for this drug. It is a low dose of the same drug (Finasteride) that is used to treat enlarged prostate glands. One of its effects is to artificially lower levels of PSA (prostate-specific antibody), a chemical in the blood that can be raised in men who are developing prostate cancer. Blood tests to check PSA levels are therefore necessary before starting treatment with Propecia to ensure that there are no problems with the prostate gland which Propecia would then mask. The treatment works well on men with early balding and also on some post-menopausal women with specific types of balding; as with Rogaine (above), it seems to be more effective on the crown and areas behind the frontal hairline. It is not recommended for younger fertile women since it can pose a risk to babies in subsequent pregnancies.

- Some people benefit greatly from the modern types of micrografting hair transplantation which, depending on the technique, can give permanent safe hair restoration. However, not everybody is a candidate. It is ideal for people who are experiencing hair loss mainly around the front of the scalp and where there is sufficient hair available for obtaining the hair grafts from the back of the head. People with fine, light hair, in particular, can respond extremely well to their hair transplant and the results are very natural. A good hair transplant, resulting in an attractive restoration of hair framing the face, can prolong a youthful and attractive appearance.

When consulting a hair transplant surgeon, you must always look into their skills and qualifications and also make sure that you are eligible for the procedure before going ahead. Ask relevant questions about issues such as side effects, the recovery period and how much improvement you can expect.

It is also important to understand that even with a successful hair transplant using micrograft techniques, you will not regain your previous hair density (say as it was in your 20s) and it will take at least 12 months for full hair growth recovery to be seen following the procedure.

* * * **WARNING!** * * *

A bad hair transplant can ruin not only your day but your looks forever, leaving you with tufts of hair and obvious scarring. Beware the advertising claims of what are often very expensive but worthless hair restoration and hair-growth remedies, as well as the claims of some trichology clinics. They frequently employ unproven lotions, scalp stimulation treatments or massage. Ask for the evidence to prove the claims, and discuss if necessary with your dermatologist, ensuring that whoever is doing the transplant has all the training, qualifications and experience required.

New Hopes for the Future

There is a real hope that it may be possible to take small samples of your hair and grow these in cell culture. Work on this procedure is progressing to produce hair growth reliably in cell cultures which can then be taken and transplanted into the scalp to show hair growth (see page 142). If this research develops successfully, it will eventually allow very small skin samples to be taken and then transplanted to the scalp, which will lead to many more people with thinning or balding hair becoming eligible candidates for hair transplants.

scars and their treatment

What is a scar?

Scars are the result of the skin's repair process for wounds caused by accidents, surgery and some diseases, and as such they are a natural part of the healing process. The more the skin is damaged the longer it takes to heal and the greater the chance of a noticeable scar. Typically a scar will become more prominent at first and then gradually fade. Many actively healing scars that seem unsightly at three months may go on to heal quite satisfactorily in time.

A scar's severity will depend on its colour, its texture, its depth, its length, its width and, very importantly, on its location: for example, scars on the front of the chest and earlobes are very prone to form what we call hypertrophic (enlarged) or keloid scars. Scar formation will also be affected by age: generally younger skin makes strong repairs and tends to heal more satisfactorily than older skin. Older skin, especially skin that is also sun-damaged, can be prone to bruising and very thin, fragile scars. The skin over the angle of the jaw is tighter than skin higher up the face, for example, on the cheeks and a scar in that area can be seen more easily and is more prone to thickening and keloid formation. If a scar is depressed, i.e. saucer-shaped, as in the case of many scars following severe acne, it will be much more noticeable and will cast a shadow causing the scar to stand out against normal skin.

A scar that crosses the natural expression lines will also be much more noticeable and a scar that is wider, for example, than a wrinkle, will stand out because it is not in the naturally occurring line.

Although it is both healthy and natural, scarring can be noticeable and sometimes very unsightly; however it can often be improved with treatment.

What can be done to treat scars?

There are several techniques that can be used to minimise scars, most of which are carried out routinely by a dermatologist under local anaesthesia. Only severe scars such as those following burns over larger areas of the body require general anaesthesia and a hospital stay. The length, width or direction of the scar can be changed by a dermatologic surgeon; however, a scar can never be raised and no magic technique will return the skin to its previously uninjured appearance. The colour of a scar can be improved with a number of treatments although it is important to realise that the scar will colour as the skin ages and may need to be camouflaged with makeup.

The first step in the treatment of scars is the consultation with the dermatologist. Each scar is different and will require a different approach. Scars need to be examined for position, type and colour and a medical history will need to be taken.

As already stated, and despite many claims that you may read in advertisements and the popular press, you cannot eliminate scars altogether. However, with the correct treatment you can reduce them, although over-treatment can lead to further damage.

• Prescription creams

Some of the most frequently used methods of scar reduction are prescription creams that contain a variety of vitamin A-related ingredients such as Tretinoin (Retin-A), Tazarotenic Acids (Tazarotene). You should also protect the scar from the sun with daily sunscreen.

Best for: minor scars.

Disadvantages: some people may experience skin irritation with some treatments such as Retin-A cream. (See also chapter 3.)

• Covers, tapes and patches

Some tapes and band-aid plaster-like devices that contain silicon have been claimed to accelerate the healing of thick scars. I am not convinced of this, having seen research that suggests that covering scars with tapes that do not contain silicon has the same benefit.

Best for: early small raised scars.

Disadvantages: experts have not seen much evidence to show that they are effective. However, they can't hurt and, compared to some of the more costly treatments, they are cheap enough to be worth a try, perhaps even in conjunction with other treatments.

- *Cortisone creams, injections and tape*

One of the most common ways used by dermatologists to reduce thick scars is to inject cortisone or to prescribe cortisone creams. These work by reducing the amount of collagen that is produced by the scar cells (fibroblasts). However, always ensure that your dermatologist has had experience in using these treatments; if a cortisone injection is too strong or too deep the result will be a scar that is depressed and the skin can become very red with spider veins. The same is true of cortisone creams and it is vital that the correct strength is prescribed.

Best for: raised red scars (hypertrophic) but also effective in shrinking and flattening larger firmer red scars (keloids).

Disadvantages: over time, cortisone can cause thinning of the skin.

(See also chapter 3.)

- *Scar subcision and surgical elevation*

This is a procedure that involves cutting under a scar with a minute blade to free the fibres of scar tissue under the skin. It is particularly useful in treating sunken, hollow scars such as those resulting from acne and chicken pox, for example.

Best for: scars on visible areas such as the face, but it is only helpful for saucer-shaped sunken scars.

Disadvantages: there is a risk of temporarily worsening the scarring; the treatment needs to be repeated.

- *Pulsed dye lasers and pulsed light sources*

These are explained in more detail on pages 58–72. They are extremely effective for treating some types of red, inflamed and thickened scars. They work by reducing the amount of blood flow through to the scar while at the same time also reducing the amount of activity of the scar tissue.

Best for: hypertrophic, red and raised scars; it is often the only practical treatment for multiple red raised scars from acne and surgery.

Disadvantages: can lead to temporary bruising; several treatments may be needed to achieve the maximum benefit.

(See also chapter 3.)

• *Microdermabrasion and chemical peels*

In this treatment superficial particles and acid solutions are applied to the skin to remove the top layers, thereby stimulating new tissue growth.

Best for: small superficial and discoloured scars to improve the skin surface quality and even out the skin tone.

Disadvantages: light peels have very little effect while deeper peels may cause redness and irritation; similarly, light microdermabrasion has little effect, while deeper microdermabrasion can cause bruising and irritation. Careful treatment is needed if you are prone to keloid scars.

(See also chapter 3.)

• *Laser resurfacing and/or dermabrasion*

This is the method by which the top layers of the skin are removed from over the scar, thus improving the surface texture and colour of the scar.

Best for: only slightly raised scars and some sunken scars where it is possible to even out the skin's surface around the scars.

Disadvantages: several treatments may be needed for deeper scars and there is a risk of increasing keloid or thickened scars. Treatment often needs to be combined with cortisone and retinoid creams to achieve good results.

(See also chapter 3.)

• *Fat injections*

The fat injected is obtained from the lower stomach or thighs using a technique called fat harvesting. It is then processed and stored in controlled conditions. Repeat treatments, together with scar subcision, are used to fill the scars and lift the surrounding skin surface.

Best for: people who have allergies to other skin fillers.

Disadvantages: several repeat treatments are often required, depending on the size of the scar.

Key facts on scarring

• Consultation with a dermatologist or plastic surgeon is vital to establish the best treatment to use.

• It is not possible to remove a scar completely, but some can be significantly improved.

• Over-treating scars or choosing the wrong treatment can actually cause further damage.

• Skin filler injections

Skin fillers (e.g. Perlane, NewFill, see pages 79–84) can be injected into sunken scars such as those that result from acne and chicken pox.

Best for: areas of sunken scars; generally impractical for very large areas such as the chest and trunk.

Disadvantages: not suitable for people with allergies to skin fillers. Also some skin fillers only last a few months while others can be longer lasting but carry certain risks (see pages 82–83).

Another filler that can be used is your own fat and this has the advantage of not having any risk of allergy (see opposite page).

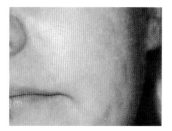

Sunken scars can be improved by NewFill, but they usually need several treatments.

• Surgical removal

This is the excision or scalpel removal of a thickened scar.

Best for: thick, wide or long scars occurring as a result of surgical procedures.

Disadvantages: it is a form of further surgery and a larger or thicker scar can result.

Summary

- It is not possible to remove a scar completely, but most scars can be improved and their appearance minimised.

- The appropriate treatment can only be assessed by a dermatological surgeon or plastic surgeon.

- There are encouraging new treatments, e.g. NewFill, the Cooltouch laser (pages 66–67) and resurfacing lasers (pages 68–72) as well as creams such as Retin-A and Tazarotene (pages 107–110) that can help to reduce some scars.

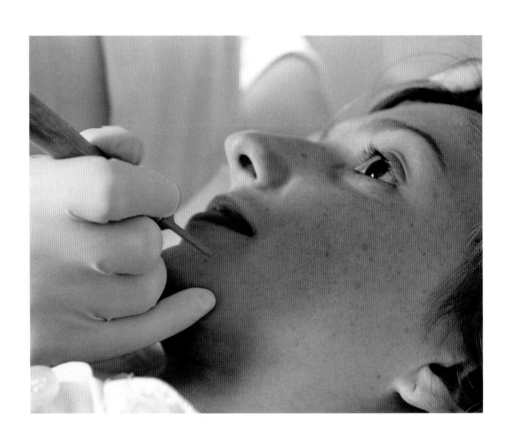

chapter three

the menu of treatments

Facial rejuvenation is a truly exciting area in which treatments that were unimaginable just ten years ago are constantly evolving and improving.

The menu of treatments is vast and can be confusing and often misleading for people who want to make improvements to their facial appearance but who are not equipped with the information they need to make an informed decision. Choosing a practitioner can be an equally daunting task, as there are many different options including dermatologists, cosmetic and dermatologic surgeons, nurses and aestheticians. This will be covered in more detail in the Appendix (see page 144) but, needless to say, both treatments and practitioners can be extremely varied in their success rate.

It is therefore essential to ensure that before you embark on any sort of cosmetic treatment or surgical procedure you know exactly what it is that you hope to achieve and that you have realistic expectations as to the likely outcome. It is also important to give yourself some sort of deadline by which you need the results of your treatment to be in place.

Again this will be covered in more detail in the Appendix (see page 144), but one of the keys to success is ensuring that you are given as much information as possible regarding all options before making up your mind about whether or not and how to proceed.

All sorts of things can lead to you taking those first tentative steps towards facial rejuvenation. There may be a school or college reunion coming up for which you would like to look your best when meeting up with old colleagues. Comments that friends or workmates have made about your appearance may have precipitated you to take action. Or you may know someone who has undergone some sort of facial

✽ Before you take any action, make sure you do the following: ✽

- Identify exactly what it is about your appearance that makes you unhappy.

- Find out about all the safe and effective procedures that can help to solve the problem/s.

- Ask as many questions as you wish. Be wary of any physician, surgeon or beauty therapist who attempts to dismiss your questions or concerns.

- Take your time during a consultation and, if you feel it necessary, seek further consultations until you are satisfied that you are in a position to make an informed decision on your treatment.

- Make sure you have information and lots of it! You need to know about the negative facts, such as side effects, as well as the positive.

- Ask to see examples of previous patients treated and, if at all possible, try to talk to some of these people about their experiences. Patients at my clinic have been happy to discuss their own past treatments with other prospective patients.

- Be honest and realistic as to your hopes and concerns about the procedure.

- **Above all, choose your cosmetic dermatologist and cosmetic surgeon very carefully** (see Appendix, page 144).

rejuvenation treatment and who now looks much younger as a result. Major life events such as divorce or bereavement are also common trigger factors.

Different problems obviously require different treatment, and different treatments work at different levels of your skin. People with mainly surface skin damage such as fine lines, sunspots and thread veins, for example, will benefit from superficial treatments such as chemical peels, microdermabrasion and the use of different lasers. Others, with deeper lines and scars that have become indented, or where fat has been lost from the middle part of their face, will need deeper treatments such as the newer, safe skin-filling agents. For more intense lines in the face caused by muscle activity and to correct brow droop, Botox can be extremely beneficial.

I will now review all the treatment options in detail, starting with the surface treatments, then moving on later to the correction of deeper problems.

chemical peels

There has been a veritable explosion of interest in chemical peeling of the skin over the last 20 years. Before the advent of resurfacing lasers, we would frequently use some of the stronger chemical peels to try to erase deeper lines. When carried out by experts the results for these strong peels could be excellent. However there was a real risk that the deeper the peel, the more white skin discolouration would occur, often leading to a patchy and irregular end product, and in some cases white and red scarring.

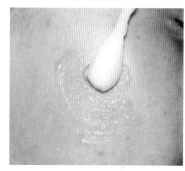

A glycolic acid peel can treat acne and sunspots.

Now, however, in the current peel revolution, we have the benefit of peels that have a much more superficial effect. To achieve optimum results, they may be repeated up to three to four times, then again annually to maintain the improvements to the skin. The focus in this book will be on superficial peels.

What is chemical peeling?

Chemical peeling involves the application to the skin of a chemical that causes a shedding of the surface skin layers. By shedding these layers, a new skin layer is formed which is both healthier and less mottled. As well as prompting this process of regrowth, the chemical also 'tricks' the dermis (the skin's supporting structure) into producing new collagen under the skin surface.

There are several types of superficial (surface) chemical peel:

- Lactic acid peels   Most superficial

- Glycolic acid peels

- Beta-hydroxy acid peels

- Jessner's peels

- Combinations of the above peels   Deeper

Medium-depth peels

Although these are beyond the scope of this book, it is useful to touch on what they are and how they compare with the surface peels. Examples of medium-depth peels include various strengths of trichloroacetic acid solution (or TCA). A lower strength of TCA, for example 10–25 per cent, could actually be used for a superficial peel, whereas a strength of 35 per cent will constitute a medium to deeper peel. These deeper peels are still used by some dermatologists, but many have moved over to laser resurfacing (see page 68) because of its potential for good control of depth.

New peels that claim to be improved types of TCA include a coloured TCA peel, along with various TCA-containing face masks. I tend to believe that these are not worthwhile improvements and that they fall into the marketing gimmick category. They are no more effective, nor are they safer than conventional TCA peels.

Preparing the skin for chemical peeling

Preparing the skin using Retin-A cream or Tazarotene cream at night or, in more olive skins, with skin-lightening agents such as pharmaceutical strengths of hydroquinone (4–5 per cent) in combination with Retin-A, is essential to the success of a chemical peel. You should use these plus a sunscreen every morning for at least six weeks before treatment for optimum results.

Glycolic acid peels

The most frequently used alpha-hydroxy acid peel is the glycolic acid peel. Glycolic acid is derived from sugar cane and is non-toxic. It is not absorbed into the body and therefore will not cause any internal side effects.

Glycolic acid stays in the outer skin layers and loosens the dead surface skin cells to reveal brighter, smoother, younger-looking skin beneath. It also helps to reduce a build-up of tired or dead cells in the upper levels of the skin. The peel promotes a healthy, youthful glow by reducing the visible signs of ageing, smoothing the complexion, balancing irregular skin tones and generally softening the skin. Research studies have confirmed that repeat glycolic acid peels of the correct strength increase skin thickness and reduce abnormal skin pigmentation.

The depth of the glycolic acid peel is controlled by three factors. These are:

- the type of glycolic acid preparation used (lotion, liquid, gel) and its ingredients

- the concentration and acidity of the glycolic acid. Aestheticians are generally restricted to using the much milder peels (25 per cent), while it is usual for dermatologists to use a concentration of 50–99 per cent. The acidity is determined by whether or not the peel has been partly neutralised by agents such as bicarbonate – in other words, the less neutralised the peel, the higher its acidity and therefore the greater its effect on your skin

- very importantly, the length of time it is left on the skin. The longer it is left, the further it penetrates and the stronger its effect (sometimes too strong on some skin types).

Your physician or their medical assistant should apply the glycolic acid and observe the skin very closely to see signs of early reddening. At your first glycolic acid peel, the glycolic acid action is stopped usually after two to four minutes by the application of cold water solution. Question your practitioner closely before starting about the type of peel they plan to use. If you are at all concerned you should insist on trying the peel on a small test area before proceeding.

It is possible to treat several areas with these peels although the most common are the face and neck. Repeat glycolic acid peels can also be quite useful for mild surface sun damage on the chest, hands and forearms.

The glycolic acid peel is generally repeated every two to four weeks for up to four to six treatments. After this, depending on how sun-damaged your skin is, a maintenance peel may be performed every month or another possibility would be to continue by using a rejuvenating cream such as Retin-A or Tazarotene.

Before, during and after treatment with glycolic acid peels

Before

Avoid any changes to your normal facial skin-care routine for one week before the peel (for example, facial hair bleaching, exfoliation, electrolysis, waxing, sunbathing and the use of tanning beds or any new creams). You must inform your physician or medical aesthetician if you do change your routine at any time during the course of treatment as this may affect your skin's response to the peel.

Your face will be cleansed with a degreasing cleanser to remove the skin's protective oil. This also allows for a better, more uniform penetration of the glycolic acid into the skin.

During

When the glycolic acid is applied you will experience a mild stinging sensation and a cooling fan will be blown on to your skin to help to alleviate this. The acid is left in place for between two and ten minutes (the time is usually increased with each treatment) before being washed off with water.

Your face will become pink after the solution is applied and then removed and there may also be some slightly whitish areas where the peel has penetrated beyond that skin but this should last only a few days.

Length of procedure: around 30 minutes (the peel takes between 2 and 10 minutes).

After

You may not actually observe any obvious shedding or peeling after the peel; however, the skin will have been stimulated to turn over more rapidly and there will be some fine scaling. If there is a blotchy appearance following the peel, this is only temporary and usually fades within a day. Light makeup may be applied immediately following the peel and you may go straight back to work if desired.

If you have small cysts (milia) or black- or whiteheads, after the peel is a good time for the medical aesthetician to remove them gently using steam and extraction.

Glycolic acid peel aftercare

- You will be advised to clean your face using a gentle, soap-free cleanser such as Aquanil or Cetaphil in the USA, or Cetaphil, pH 5.5 or Dermol 500 lotion in the UK. This is important in helping to prevent any increased drying of the skin. It also boosts your skin's tolerance to subsequent peels and creams such as Retin-A.

- Moisturisers may be applied to the face twice a day, again to improve the skin's tolerance to further treatment.

- Sunscreen should be applied each morning (see page 112).

- If you notice some visible peeling do not be tempted to pick at or peel the dead peeling skin as this may increase the risk of discolouration. Use an effective moisturiser (e.g. Cetaphil cream, Eucerin, Nivea, Neutrogena, Neostrata moisturising cream or Vaseline facial moisturiser) to smooth the peeling skin.

- If you experience any unusual reactions, such as excessive blotchiness or irregular shedding, it is most important that you contact your practitioner.

Possible complications of glycolic acid peels

- Some patients may experience more pain and stinging than others, especially those with sensitive skin types or eczema sufferers, for example. This usually resolves once the glycolic acid is washed off but if the stinging is too severe you must consult your practitioner so that they can reduce the strength and duration of the peel at the next session.

- Temporary brown discolouration may occur in some patients after a peel, despite efforts to avoid sun exposure. Sunscreens and skin lightening creams can minimise these effects. In a small percentage (less than 1 per cent) a permanent change of skin colour can occur.

- Some acne spots may become temporarily more red and noticeable.

- People with a herpes simplex virus history (cold sores or fever blisters) may find that symptoms are brought on by the peel. It is therefore important to tell your physician in advance of treatment if you are prone to this so that they can prescribe appropriate medication (e.g. Acyclovir tablets) to prevent it. I would routinely prescribe a low dose of Acyclovir to be taken daily throughout a course of peels for anyone who has a history of fever blisters or cold sores.

Beta-hydroxy acid peels

These are varying concentrations of salicylic acid (related to the chemical in aspirin) in a peel. They are similar to the glycolic acid peels in most ways, the main difference being that these are slightly stronger and may cause more redness and surface peeling. They have many uses for the skin including shedding warts and helping acne.

They are generally recommended for more severely sun-damaged skin or for more serious acne or spots. Salicylic acid peels work well in acne-prone skin but are not advisable for very sensitive skin types. It is also possible to start a patient with glycolic acid peels and, if they are tolerating these well, move on to the salicylic acid variety.

For more detailed information regarding preparation for treatment, the treatment itself (lasting 50–55 minutes) and possible complications, see glycolic acid peels (pages 50–53). You can go straight back to work after treatment and a moisturiser and light makeup may be applied immediately.

Glycolic, beta-hydroxy and lactic acid peels: what they can and cannot do

Can help:

- superficial discolouration
- superficial blemishes and scars
- smaller acne spots
- fine lines
- to promote a healthy glow by reducing build-up of dead cells in outer skin layers
- blackheads and whiteheads

Cannot help:

- severe discolouration
- prominent scars from past acne, for example
- thread veins
- deeper lines

Lactic acid peels

Lactic acid is another of the alpha-hydroxy acid peels obtained originally from milk and dairy products. Lactic acid peels are extremely valuable for people with very sensitive skin. They are often used successfully in patients for whom it is neither possible nor practical to use glycolic or salicylic acids due to their skin's sensitivity. Lactic acid peels are usually well tolerated and lead to less peeling and skin shredding than glycolic and beta peels. Lactic acid could be considered an 'entry level' peel.

For more detailed information regarding preparation for treatment, the treatment itself (lasting up to 30 minutes) and possible complications, see glycolic acid peels (pages 50–53). You may go straight back to work after treatment.

Jessner's solution peels

These are a combination of chemicals in a peel, named after the American dermatologist who formulated it. This peel contains salicylic acid, lactic acid and resorcinol (another skin-peeling chemical) which together constitute a very adjustable peel which lends itself well to repeat applications.

It is similar in most ways to the glycolic acid peel (see pages 50–53), but there are certain important differences.

Jessner's peels can be applied in varying amounts to different areas at one session, depending on the area of skin to be treated and the amount of damage or ageing sustained. For example, there may be mild to moderate damage on a patient's face and chest but only mild damage on the neck. In such a case I would apply three to five coats to the face and chest (i.e. the more damaged and tougher areas of skin) but probably only two to the neck, where the damage is less serious and the skin is more delicate.

Another benefit of the Jessner's peels is that they can be used on areas such as the neck, chest, arms and hands and occasionally the legs if there is surface skin damage. The results will always be better if good pre-peel treatment has been performed (see box on page 50).

Jessner's peels cause some redness for one to two days after treatment, often similar in appearance to very mild sunburn. Several days later there will be some fine surface peeling in the areas treated.

Jessner's peels can be repeated safely many times over the course of several years to achieve and maintain a good level of rejuvenation.

For more detailed information regarding preparation for treatment, the treatment itself (lasting 30–60 minutes) and possible complications, see glycolic acid peels (pages 50–53). You may apply makeup and return to work straight after treatment but your face will be slightly pink.

In conclusion

The superficial peels detailed above are generally my most frequently used peels. My specific choice of peel is based on the patient's skin type, history of skin sensitivity and the areas of skin to be peeled. I tend to use modern laser resurfacing (see pages 68–72) for treating more sun-damaged faces, in preference to stronger peels such as TCA.

* * * Contraindications * * *

Superficial chemical peels are safe except in cases where a patient has a history of cold sores (herpes simplex) on the face in which case a course of anti-herpes simplex tablets would be prescribed. After these peels, sunscreens should be used to avoid skin pigment changes in olive and darker skins.

microdermabrasion

Microdermabrasion is a relatively recent process that has gained in popularity over the last five to ten years. It is a system in which very small crystals (such as aluminium salts, sodium chloride or sodium bicarbonate) are sucked across the surface of the skin causing the removal of the surface skin cells – hence 'micro-derm-abrasion'.

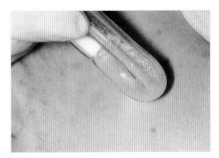

Microdermabrasion treatment.

In fact my own research group in California studied one of the early microdermabrasion machines manufactured in Italy about 20 years ago, but at that time I felt it was neither powerful nor consistent enough to be of value. Since that time, however, major refinements in the machines and in the techniques employed for microdermabrasion have made it a much more useful form of treatment.

In general, the more powerful machines are made available to dermatologists and other physicians, while the less powerful machines are used by beauty therapists and aestheticians.

Microdermabrasion has been shown to be particularly beneficial when used in conjunction with glycolic acid chemical peels (see pages 50–53) and topical creams such as Retin-A and skin-lightening combinations (see pages 107–110) for problems such as facial pigmentation (such as dark skin or mask of pregnancy).

Microdermabrasion: what it can and cannot do

Can help:

- areas of whiteheads, blackheads and small acne spots
- dark, superficial scars
- irregular pigmentation
- small shallow scars
- to brighten dull skin, making it more vital and alive

Cannot help:

- deeper, more serious scarring (hypertrophic or keloid scars)
- spider or thread veins
- lumps on the skin
- deeper levels of dark patches

Microdermabrasion is usually given at least once or twice a month.

Before, during and after treatment with microdermabrasion

Before

No special skin preparation is required other than cleansing with gentle, soap-free cleansers.

During

You will feel a very superficial scraping, similar to a loofah or a mild skin exfoliation.

Length of procedure: session lasts for between 30 minutes (for the face) and 60 minutes (for the face, neck and chest).

After

You can go out and about and makeup may be applied immediately after treatment, if desired. There should be no soreness but your skin may look brighter and pinker straight after treatment.

Microdermabrasion treatment aftercare

As for glycolic acid peel aftercare, see pages 52–53.

Possible complications

Microdermabrasion may be used on all types and there should be no visible problems if it is correctly performed, other than a slight pinkness of the skin on the face or hands immediately after the session. However, if the treatment has been carried out too deeply, there can be surface skin bruising and a change of colour. These problems usually resolve themselves quickly except in the case of olive or darker skin types (phototypes 3, 4, 5 and 6 – see pages 28–29) in which the pigmentation can be more severe and longer lasting.

*   Contraindications   *

As for chemical peels, page 55.

lasers

Lasers for Skin Discolouration and Pigmentation

The first laser to be used in medicine, in the early 1960s, was called the Ruby laser and was developed by the pioneering American dermatologist, the late Leon Goldman who was still carrying out laser research in his 90s. Dr Goldman found that the Ruby laser was highly effective at reducing the colour of tattoos and some brown pigment spots, although others learned that there was less of a risk of incurring skin damage when short-pulsed and Q-switched lasers were developed.

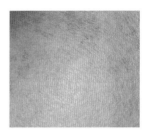

Sunspots on the cheek are excellent candidates for removal by the Q-switch Ruby laser.

Short-pulsed lasers

A modification to the Ruby laser, which makes it deliver very high bursts of energy in a fraction of a second (known as Q-switching) has made it much safer, so that it is now used routinely for the removal of darker tattoos and sunspots, as well as some brown or blue birthmarks and dark pigmentation circles under the eyes.

Other related Q-switched lasers used for brown pigmentation and tattoos include the Q-switched Alexandrite laser which goes slightly deeper than the Ruby laser, and the Q-switched Nd: YAG laser, which goes deeper still and can treat red tattoos.

Q-switched lasers: what they can and cannot do

Can help:

- blue/green/black tattoos (Ruby) and red tattoos (Nd: YAG)
- sunspots (lentigo)
- dark circles under the eyes
- some dark scars
- some **benign*** birthmarks

Cannot help:

- some darker skin types (phototypes 3–6, see pages 28–29) as a loss of pigmentation may occur in some cases (a skin test should be performed on a small area as a precaution)
- brown or black moles

* **Note:** pigmented moles should always be checked by a dermatologist to ensure that they are benign; lasers should never be used on an undiagnosed mole. Often a biopsy is needed to be certain.

Longer-pulsed pigment lasers: what they can and cannot do

Can help:

- biopsy-proven benign moles
- certain birthmarks, such as some *café au lait* brown patches
- many types of excess skin hair growth

Cannot help:

- some darker skin types (phototypes 4–6, see page 29) as permanent discolouration can result

Longer-pulsed lasers

Once it was discovered that the Q-switched lasers were effective for treating sun-spots and tattoos, but that they were less so for biopsy-proven benign moles and hair removal, the next step was to extend the pulse duration. Other safe lasers for the removal of brown spots and pigment were developed. The result was known as long-pulsed or normal-pulsed Ruby, Alexandrite or Nd: YAG lasers. This has given us lasers that can remove hair and treat proven benign moles and brown birthmarks.

Before, during and after laser treatment for skin discolouration

Before

If you have olive or darker skin or a suntan, special precautions need to be taken before this form of treatment. In such cases a lightening cream and sunscreen should be used in order to prevent the laser from being absorbed by the tan. Some people with dark skin may not be suitable for this treatment.

During

You will be required to wear laser-protective goggles. The laser physician targets the skin area to be treated and activates the laser. A skin-pricking or snapping sensation is felt. If this is uncomfortable, you will be offered a local anaesthetic cream.

Length of procedure: this depends on the area being treated – for areas on the face allow up to an hour; for a hand, allow 15–30 minutes.

After

Some crusting and weeping may occur but should mostly heal quickly over a three-to-four-day period. Some tattoo treatments may take longer to heal. You may return to work immediately after treatment and if it is your face that has been treated you may apply makeup to camouflage any temporary skin discolouration.

You will be given band-aids or non-stick dressings as well as antibiotic ointments or creams to be used for up to four to five days. Use a sunscreen once dressings have been removed. If you have been treated for sunspots or brown birthmarks, you should be given a skin-lightening cream to use for a week.

Possible complications

Scarring can occur (particularly with some tattoos) or loss of pigment. Results may be poor with some darker birthmarks.

Blood Vessel Lasers for Thread Veins, Red Birthmarks and Red Faces

Two American dermatologists, Dr Rox Anderson and Professor John Parish, developed a laser similar to the Q-switched laser in that it delivers short bursts of energy in a short period, but designed specifically to treat blood vessel disorders. This short-pulsed laser produces a yellow light that is absorbed very efficiently by the red colour (haemoglobin) in the enlarged blood vessels of red and purple birthmarks, and, as it was discovered following further research, spider veins and other forms of redness, such as rosacea.

Longer-pulsed lasers have since been developed for blood vessels. One of the very latest is one that I use in my London practice, which has the advantage of being able to vary the length of time taken for the laser light to be delivered. In practical terms this means it can be adjusted for larger or smaller blood vessels. Also, interestingly, whereas the short-pulsed blood vessel lasers caused a bruising discolouration which could last up to seven to ten days, with longer-pulsed lasers this side effect can be minimised.

The most common type of facial blood vessel abnormality is the spider vein or thread vein, which occurs largely as a result of hereditary factors, hormonal factors (in pregnancy, for example), sunlight, accelerated skin ageing, local injury to the skin and repetitive flushing or blushing (with or without the rosacea – see page 36).

Blood vessel lasers: what they can and cannot do

Can help:

- spider or thread veins, especially on face and upper body, or very small thread veins on the legs
- blood vessel birthmarks
- to improve (but possibly not clear) some facial flushing and rosacea
- red acne spots
- to improve hypertrophic or keloid scars (these require multiple treatments)
- to improve fine lines in pink skin

Cannot help:

- any red spots that may not be benign*
- some leg veins, particularly large blue ones
- severe facial flushing
- some darker skin types (phototypes 3–6, see pages 28–29)

* Note: some skin cancers can be red and mistaken for enlarged blood vessel spots, so these should always be checked by a specialist dermatologist before any treatment with lasers is undertaken.

Another is the congenital birthmark, composed of greatly enlarged blood vessels in the skin and described as a haemangioma. Perhaps the most famous example of this type of birthmark is that seen on the forehead of Mikhail Gorbachev, the last president of the former Soviet Union.

Before, during and after treatment with blood vessel lasers

Before

No special preparation is required, but some dark skin types may not be suitable.

During

You will be given laser-protective goggles to protect your eyes during treatment. You will experience a sensation not unlike that of rubber bands flicking against your skin as the laser pulses the light into your skin. Newer lasers cool and anaesthetise the skin surface with cold air sprays, making it less uncomfortable.

Length of procedure: this depends on the extent of skin to be treated – the nose area will take around 10 minutes; whole lower face, 30–60 minutes.

After

You may see some darker redness or purple colour where you have been treated. Makeup may be applied immediately after treatment since the skin surface is not broken. Many people go straight back to work after treatment as the area usually looks just a little redder than before and women can normally hide this with camouflage makeup.

Blood vessel laser treatment aftercare

Sunscreen should be applied if laser treatment was on the face.

Possible complications

You should be very cautious about receiving this type of laser if you are prone to dark skin discolouration (in particular skin phototypes 3–6, see pages 28–29). In the great majority of people the red or bruising discolouration will clear after seven to ten days but, in a smaller percentage of people this can turn into dark pigmentation, particularly on the legs, that can last for many months.

Laser and Light Rejuvenation without Resurfacing (Non-ablative Skin Rejuvenation)

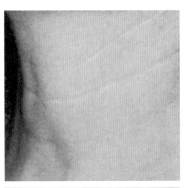

Another new, exciting development is the use of blood vessel lasers and light machines in a treatment known as non-ablative skin rejuvenation. The term 'non-ablative' is used to indicate the fact that no obvious skin surface injury is sustained (i.e. no peeling, crusting or scabbing). Instead, a variety of lasers and special light machines penetrate the skin surface and cause the blood vessels to release growth factors that stimulate new collagen in the skin. Fine lines and mild to moderate sun damage may be improved as a result, and surface abnormalities such as thread veins and brown spots may also benefit.

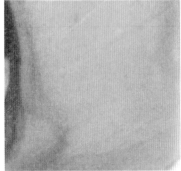

Fine lines on the face and neck can be safely and conveniently treated during your lunchbreak.

A variety of lasers and light systems is used for non-ablative rejuvenation, all of them based on the premise of increasing collagen production. They are:

- intense pulsed light (IPL) systems

- blood vessel pulsed dye lasers

- long wavelength lasers (absorbed by the skin's water content)

Intense pulsed light (IPL) rejuvenation (photofacial or photorejuvenation)

Also sometimes known as a flash lamp, IPL systems work by being absorbed by the skin surface abnormalities and also by the superficial thread veins and normal veins in the skin. This process releases growth factors that produce new collagen. It is also thought that they work by heating the skin below the surface, again to produce more collagen by stimulating the cells called fibroblasts. A non-laser light source is used and various filters are used with it to remove the shorter 'harmful' wavelengths. I now routinely use one of these systems (a Lumenis IPL system) in my London practice.

Treatment with IPL can be very effective for lighter-skinned (skin phototypes 1, 2 and some type 3, see page 28) patients in particular, although often between three and five treatment sessions are required. It may also be necessary to have further courses of treatment every one or two years to maintain improvements. IPL treatment can damage pigmentation in people with darker skin (phototypes 5–6, see page 29) so it is always best to ask for treatment to be carried out on a small test area first. Treatment on phototypes 3 and 4 is possible, but I use different energy settings from those I would use on types 1 and 2.

IPL: what it can and cannot do

Can help:

- dull-looking skin
- mild flushing
- patchy brown sunspots
- thread veins
- fine lines

Cannot help:

- severe skin damage such as deep wrinkles and sagging skin
- severe flushing
- some darker skin types (phototypes 5–6, see page 29)

Before, during and after treatment with IPL

Before

A lightening cream and sunscreen may be used before treatment if patients have olive skin or a suntan. Also, patients who have a history of herpes simplex may be prescribed anti-virus medication as well as oral antibiotics prior to treatment. A local anaesthetic cream is sometimes used, as mild to moderate discomfort may be experienced during treatment.

During

A cooled gel is applied to the skin to help reduce pain and also the risk of skin blistering. The IPL causes a snapping sensation against the skin as the light is released into the skin by the machine.

Length of procedure: between 45 minutes (whole face) and 1 hour (face and neck).

After

There will be a mild redness in the areas treated. You should be able to apply makeup and return to work immediately after treatment.

IPL treatment aftercare

After treatment with IPL it is most important that you continue to protect your skin with sunscreen and a maintenance rejuvenation cream such as Retin-A, as well as topical vitamin C creams (see chapter 4).

Possible complications

Some skin discolouration can occur (both increased and decreased pigmentation) if incorrect energy settings are used – as always ensure that your physician or medical assistant is fully trained.

Occasionally, if your skin is redder than usual (due to mild sun exposure or heat), it may absorb more of the light and your skin will temporarily turn a dark red or bruised colour for up to ten days. Very rare cases of scarring have been reported.

Blood Vessel Lasers as Non-ablative Rejuvenating Systems

The blood vessel pulsed dye lasers developed to treat port-wine birthmarks and thread veins (see pages 60–61) have also been used successfully in skin rejuvenation, particularly for fair skin with spider veins or background redness.

It is thought that the blood vessel lasers act in a rejuvenating capacity by causing a slight injury to the blood vessels in the skin, which then respond by releasing growth factors that stimulate the fibroblast cells in the dermis to produce new collagen.

Considerable media attention has been focused on the N-lite laser, which actually uses older technology that we had been using for many years to treat spider veins and birthmarks. Newer laser systems such as the variable pulsed blood vessel lasers (e.g. Candella and Cynosure systems) are, in fact, more effective and selective than the N-lite laser. My own clinic employs the Cynosure laser with a special skin-cooling device using refrigerated air, which I have found to be extremely beneficial for skin rejuvenation, spider veins, red birthmarks, some red facial treatments and treatment of inflamed acne spots.

Treatment should be either carried out or closely supervised by a laser dermatologist and care must be taken to avoid developing blotchy patches within existing areas of brown or red discolouration. These may subsequently show up as 'over-treated' whiter patches. Second or third treatments may be needed to achieve a uniform result.

Before, during and after rejuvenation treatment with blood vessel lasers

Before

No special preparation, but any suntan should be allowed to fade before treatment.

During

You will feel a cold air spray and a slight pricking sensation as the laser fires.

Length of procedure: between 30 minutes (for the lower half of the face) and 1 hour (for face and neck). Usually several treatments are required.

After

Your face may be very slightly pink for one to two days, but you may return to work immediately.

Possible complications

Red patches of discolouration can occur but usually last only for a few days and camouflage makeup may be used to disguise these if necessary.

Longer wavelength lasers for rejuvenation

The longer wavelength lasers that I discussed on page 59 (e.g. different types of YAG lasers) can also be used to improve fine lines and surface mottling, again, it is thought, by helping to stimulate new collagen under the skin by heating the fibroblasts. The Cooltouch system and the Smoothbeam lasers are both effective for this type of treatment. The laser energy is absorbed by the water content of the skin.

Before, during and after treatment with long-pulsed lasers

Before

No special preparation is required. All skin types (phototypes 1–6, see pages 28–29) can be treated.

Cooltouch and Smoothbeam lasers: what they can and cannot do

Can help:

- all skin types
- fine lines
- fine scars
- some stretch marks

Cannot help:

- more severe ageing
- loose or lax skin
- thread veins
- red face patches
- brown patches

During

More pain is likely to be experienced with these types of laser because the skin is heated quite deeply. This can be overcome by the application of anaesthetic creams before the lasers are used. You will feel a sharp snapping sensation, rather like a rubber band flicking on the skin.

Length of procedure: up to 30 minutes for the face; up to 1 hour for face and neck.

After

There may be slight redness but you can return to work immediately after treatment. Makeup may be applied straight away. There should be no post-laser pain.

Possible complications

The long-pulsed laser systems (e.g. Cooltouch and Smoothbeam) have to be cooled very efficiently in order to protect the skin surface from heat blisters, but if the cooling spray itself is not delivered at the correct time, it can lead to cold-induced blisters instead. Also, if the laser is used at too high a setting it may cause skin burns and subsequent discolouration.

laser resurfacing

Laser resurfacing involves, in the optimum situation, the controlled removal of layers of sun- or scar-damaged skin, allowing the body to replace them with more youthful and less scarred skin. Performed correctly, this procedure has several advantages over treatments such as mechanical dermabrasion, where it is more difficult to achieve a uniform effect on the whole face. (Mechanical dermabrasion is more aggressive than microdermabrasion and uses small electric skin abraders.) It is also much more controlled than the deeper chemical peels such as the higher strength TCA peels (see page 50).

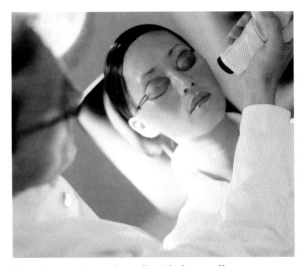

The ultra-pulse carbon dioxide laser offers natural facial rejuvenation.

Unfortunately, however, media hype and encouragement from the laser companies initially attracted many specialists and non-specialists who lacked suitable training. In some cases they have been 'trained' at weekend courses and often their treatment has led to scarring and skin discolouration. It is essential, therefore, to ensure that this form of treatment is carried out only by someone who has been fully and appropriately trained in its use. Ask to see certificates of training in the use of these lasers, and also to speak to and see photographs of previously treated patients.

History of resurfacing lasers

In the late 1980s my colleagues, Drs Gary Lask and Larry David, in southern California, used a carbon dioxide laser to remove precancerous skin patches on the upper lip. Following the removal, during the course of healing, they noted that lines that the patient had on the upper lip were also considerably improved. This led to the first report on laser skin resurfacing, following which I worked closely with Dr Lask to select safer lasers to provide the benefits of skin resurfacing while reducing the risks of scarring and skin colour change.

Types of skin resurfacing lasers

The ultimate laser (and still my personal preference today) was developed approximately four years after these initial observations. It was the UltraPulse carbon-dioxide laser, which was produced by an American company called Coherent. This laser had special characteristics in that it allowed the delivery of energy in very small fractions of a microsecond. In practical terms this enabled an almost layer-by-layer removal of damaged skin. Also, the density or thickness of skin removal could be varied using computer-controlled delivery of the laser. Other lasers developed subsequently include the erbium:YAG lasers, which were even more precise and very versatile but did not seal the blood vessels in the way that the UltraPulse CO_2 did and therefore tended to cause considerable bleeding. (There is now an erbium:YAG laser that can 'copy' the benefits of the UltraPulse carbon-dioxide laser.)

It has become apparent that by doing more superficial skin resurfacing it is possible to achieve a much more rapid healing process than is possible with deeper, more aggressive laser treatment. As a result of this, patients are often able to return to work eight or nine days after the procedure. This technique is much less severe than the old one, following which it could frequently take several weeks, if not months, for the patient's skin to return to normal. It also allows for follow-up treatment to take place 12 months or so later to attain further improvement.

Another advantage of the more superficial modern technique that I now use is that patients with olive or darker skin (phototypes 3–6, see pages 28–29) can be successfully treated without loss of pigment, scarring or mottling, which were risks inherent in the old technique. The superficial approach is also excellent for the treatment of the face and neck, as it means that you are not left with a line of changed skin at the jaw and, as a result, the neck skin blends in nicely with the facial skin.

To determine the success of skin rejuvenation and scar treatment the ultimate test is how the skin looks a year after treatment. The best results in the majority of cases seemed to be with the UltraPulse carbon-dioxide laser, and one of our studies showed that when the degree of skin improvement was followed every month for a year, the improvement at 12 months was considerably greater than it had been at 2 or 3 months.

The delayed improvement occurs because after the surface skin has been removed by the laser, the skin is then stimulated to produce a new external layer or epidermis. In addition, the dermis is stimulated to produce a larger number of active cells (fibroblasts) which, in turn, prompt the production of new collagen and elastin. These are laid down gradually over the 12 months following the laser treatment and it is this that causes a steady tightening of the face, improvement of skin quality, elasticity and filling and tightening of facial scars.

Before, during and after treatment with laser resurfacing

Before
Patients should be prescribed oral anti-herpes simplex virus medication prior to undergoing laser resurfacing treatment, as well as oral antibiotics.

During
Laser skin resurfacing should be performed using anaesthesia. Areas around the eyes and the upper lip can be treated with local anaesthesia creams plus injections of anaesthesia. For whole face and neck resurfacing I always work very closely with a consultant anaesthetist who administers a very short-acting sedation anaesthesia. This allows the patient to wake quickly following the procedure and to go home with a companion as little as one or two hours after treatment.

* * * **Laser skin resurfacing:
what it can and cannot do** * * *

Can help:
- moderate/severe sun damage
- multiple wrinkles extending into the cheeks, around the eyes and upper lip
- sunken acne or other scars
- multiple sunspots and benign surface skin blemishes (e.g. brown keratoses)
- mild sun damage and ageing of the neck

Cannot help:
- very deep scars (these require fillers and laser)
- sagging skin
- sagging neck
- fat bags under the eyes
- lines caused by muscle movement e.g. deep forehead lines (these need Botox before the laser)

Laser skin resurfacing: the myths and the facts

Myth You will never be able to go out in the sun again following laser skin resurfacing (see aftercare guidelines below).

Fact You can go out in the sun using an appropriate sunscreen (see pages 111–115); after all, laser skin resurfacing started life in southern California – a very sunny climate.

Myth Laser skin resurfacing will leave you with bad facial redness for many months.

Fact This used to be a possibility when treatment was administered too aggressively, but with the modern approach described on page 69, this is no longer the case.

Myth Laser resurfacing carries a high risk of skin infection.

Fact This not true, provided that the patient is treated appropriately (see 'Before', above and 'After').

The laser releases its energy into the skin surface, 'vapourising' the surface skin damage. If the skin is badly sun-damaged or wrinkled then local areas (e.g. upper lip skin) can be treated with a second laser 'pass'.

After

Immediately after treatment I apply a non-sensitising, mild moisturising ointment that the patient should then apply themselves several times a day. This is preferable to covering patients with masks which not only is unpleasant, but also provides ideal conditions for bacterial growth on the skin and skin infections. The skin will have the appearance of being severely sunburned with redness and swelling, particularly around the eyelids. The skin will then start to shed and peel after around three to five days. Between seven and ten days after treatment, it should be looking pink and smooth. There is usually no pain during this healing process, but there may be some itching.

* * * Contraindications to laser skin resurfacing * * *

This form of treatment is not recommended for people with keloid scars, anyone who has been taking RoAccutane/Accutane within the year preceding proposed treatment or anyone at risk of pigment loss as a result of a disease called vitiligo.

Laser resurfacing treatment aftercare

I examine patients every day for the first five to eight days following treatment.

Patients should give their face gentle water soaks using a clean face cloth and/or stand under a slow-running warm (not hot) shower to rinse gently the treated area/s. After each soaking or shower, they can apply a non-sensitising moisturiser as often as they like – up to every two hours. These techniques are very helpful in promoting rapid healing and excellent results.

About ten days after treatment, it is advisable to start using a broad-spectrum sunscreen (see pages 112–114) to protect the skin, and you can use a camouflage makeup covering if desired when you are in public. About four weeks after treatment, you should start using Retin-A or lightening creams (see pages 107–110) to prevent the return of dark patches. (It is best not to do this sooner as these creams can irritate recently lasered skin.)

botox

Botox is one of the types of botulinum toxin type A, often abbreviated to BTX or BXTA. It was originally developed medically in 1973 by Dr Alan Scott, an eye surgeon in San Francisco, as a non-surgical and safe way of treating a squint in children. Its use was then successfully extended to treat a condition called blepharospasm where the eyelids and other parts of the face go into a nervous tic or spasm. It was by observing Botox in this context that a husband-and-wife team (Drs Jean and Alastair Carruthers, an eye specialist and dermatologist in Canada) noted that it also reduced the wrinkles in the upper face. The rest, as they say, is history and Botox is now employed to treat upper facial lines such as crow's feet and deep vertical forehead lines caused by facial and neck muscles, using its ability to temporarily interrupt the flow of nerve messages to the muscles.

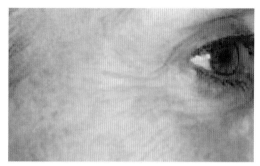

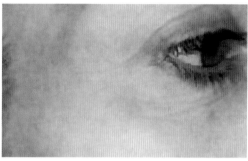

Crow's feet, caused by the smiling muscle, can be treated by Botox.

Unfortunately Botox has suffered at the hands of the media in the same way as laser resurfacing (see page 68) with the result that many of the people who use it to treat patients are not adequately trained to do so. Although, on the whole, the side effects of Botox are self-limiting and mostly wear off within four months, it is possible for the untrained physician to inject it in the wrong location, causing more serious problems, such as facial deformity, which can be very distressing for up to several weeks or even months.

If you are considering treatment with Botox, as with all other treatments, you must ensure that the person you are consulting (who should ideally be either a trained dermatologist, dermatologic surgeon, ophthalmic or plastic surgeon) has the appropriate speciality training, and always follow the general guidelines given on pages 144–153 before going ahead. Botox has enormous potential for the successful treatment of facial lines and wrinkles and it would be a great tragedy if this were to be compromised by untrained practitioners.

Botox for facial lines

Botox may be used either alone or in combination with other treatments such as light and laser rejuvenation (see pages 62–72) and skin fillers (see pages 79–85). One test that I would use to assess whether or not a patient is a suitable candidate for treatment with Botox is to observe them at rest. If lines are visible at rest and give a noticeably increased appearance of ageing of the skin or 'worry' lines, I would certainly recommend this form of treatment. If, however, they have mild, slight lines at frown and at smile but no lines at rest, I will often recommend that they wait until later to undergo Botox treatment, and use creams such as Retin-A or Tazarotene (see pages 107–110) in the interim.

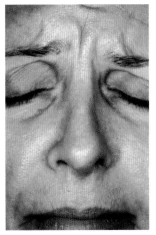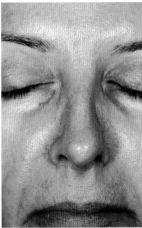

Deep central forehead lines can make you look worried or angry. See how much calmer she looks after treatment with Botox injections.

The most commonly treated upper facial lines are the vertical ones between the eyebrows and forehead, known as glabella lines. In addition, the horizontal forehead lines are also frequently treated.

Botox:
what it can and cannot do

Can help:

- lines between the eyes
- more severe horizontal forehead lines
- mild eyebrow droop
- crow's feet
- neck bands
- downturned 'sad' lips

Cannot help:

- sagging skin of face and neck
- severe dropped forehead
- thin lips
- sunspots
- surface skin blemishes
- thread veins

The glabella lines are often accompanied by drooping of the brows (see left) and Botox can have the effect of creating a significant browlift. Ideally a subtle browlift is desirable to avoid arching of the eyebrows but if overarching does occur, this can be softened and reduced by injecting very small amounts of Botox into the forehead muscle in the mid-brow area above the arching eyebrow.

Botox has a very good success rate with the lines that radiate from the outer part of the eye (crow's feet). Although the effects do not always seem to last as long as they do with treatment of the forehead muscles, with larger doses it is possible to achieve results that can last between four and six months.

In some patients the lines that run horizontally along the lower eyelids can also successfully be treated with Botox. Often, in fact, they can be made more noticeable when the crow's feet area is treated and I usually recommend that these lines are also injected using very small quantities of Botox.

Before, during and after treatment with Botox

Before

A local anaesthetic cream is administered 15 minutes before treatment. No other preparation is necessary.

During

You should feel only a tiny pinprick sensation. I always mix my Botox with a solution that numbs the skin. Tiny amounts are injected into the relevant muscles, which are identified by getting you either to frown or smile. I use the thinnest of needles.

Length of procedure: 15–20 minutes including the application of anaesthetic cream.

After

To increase the 'uptake' of the Botox you should try to use the injected muscles for about 30 minutes after treatment (i.e. smile or frown) as much as possible. Avoid massaging the area for around 24 hours. No camouflage makeup is needed and you can return to work immediately.

* **NOTE** *

All unnecessary treatments and injections should be avoided if you are, or suspect that you may be pregnant.

Botox should start to work between four and seven days after injection. If you are unhappy with the results of your treatment, you should talk to your injecting physician regarding the possibility of adjusting the effects with further smaller injections.

Botox treatment aftercare

No aftercare required.

Possible complications of Botox treatment for upper facial lines

In some patients, there is a possibility that as Botox successfully reduces activity in some muscles, others appear to become more powerful, producing new lines, most particularly above the eyebrows. Technically this is not a side effect, but a direct result of the effects of Botox on those muscles that have been targeted. It can easily be countered by giving further Botox treatment to those muscles that are creating the new lines.

Another potential problem is that if Botox is injected too far outward to the sides of the forehead, it can produce a weakening of the muscles that support the brow, thus leading to a drooping of the brow. In all cases this effect will right itself, although this can take several weeks. It is also possible to inject more Botox in very small quantities into the muscles responsible for brow depression to improve this droop. Alternatively, Botox may be injected just below the brow to cause brow elevation. These are, however, advanced techniques that should only ever be undertaken by skilled dermatologic surgeons and plastic surgeons.

Another complication that can arise very occasionally is that of temporary double vision, which can last up to six weeks. This can occur if the botulinum toxin spreads into the muscles that control eye movement but it will correct itself without further treatment. In my experience I have never actually seen this happen with Botox itself, but I have seen it with the injection of another botulinum toxin type A called Dysport, which is more prone to spread to neighbouring muscles. This suggests to me that Botox is a more precise treatment than Dysport.

Mid and lower facial lines – treatment with Botox

Botox can be used in some parts of the lower face, but special expertise by the practitioner is required to achieve the desired effect as there is a greater risk of affecting other muscles, possibly causing some paralysis of the lower face, which can last up to several months.

In the lower face, Botox can be very successful in treating lines around the lips caused by pursing (found in heavy smokers, for example) and marionette or sad lines. It can also achieve good results with the ageing neck, for example vertical bands or 'turkey neck'. These are actually muscle bands that have become visible through the loss of fat around the neck. However, this approach will only work for patients who have distinct vertical neck bands without much lax skin.

Botox versus botulinum toxin type B

A very few people develop a resistance to Botox type A and they can be treated with botulinum toxin type B (also used for the treatment of neck spasm), known as Neurobloc in Europe and as Myobloc in the USA. But how does it compare with Botox for facial lines? Studies I have carried out with my research group in the USA show the following:

- patients find treatment with type B much more painful

- the positive effects of Botox are much longer lasting (in some of our studies they have been shown to last twice as long)

- type B toxin spreads much more than Botox, which makes it virtually impossible to target the exact muscles required to achieve reduction of some localised facial lines; it also, therefore, carries a higher risk of complications such as double vision or eyelid drooping (see above)

- the localised targeting ability of Botox means it is able to achieve a much better non-surgical browlift when injected into the central forehead muscles.

My own personal preference is for Botox over Dysport or the type B toxins because there has been far more research into Botox than into the others, giving us evidence of its precision and benefits, and reassurances about its safety.

* * * Botox: the myths and the facts * * *

Myth Botox is a dangerous muscle poison.

Fact Botox injections have been used safely and effectively for over 20 years to treat many eye and neurological conditions including spasticity and cerebral palsy in children. The recommendation for the safe treatment of Botox is to ensure that you choose a registered specialist – either a certified dermatologist or plastic surgeon with special training in Botox.

Myth You should not travel by air shortly after undergoing Botox treatment.

Fact Any problems experienced when flying after Botox treatment are almost certainly due to a fault in the way the treatment was carried out rather than the combination of Botox and flying. I myself have been treated with Botox shortly before flying from the USA to the UK without experiencing any problems.

Myth Creams containing Botox-like substances can be as effective as Botox.

Fact There has recently been an explosion of inaccurate claims suggesting that creams (with names sounding mysteriously like Botox) can produce results as good as Botox itself. Botox needs to be delivered by injection into the muscles that are producing lines, e.g. forehead or smile line muscles, and cream treatments quite simply cannot do this.

In summary, Botox has proven to be a highly successful and safe form of treatment. I have carried out studies on well over a thousand patients myself in carefully controlled conditions, and have treated many more in my clinics. Several hundred thousand patients have been successfully treated worldwide with Botox. It is, in my view, the gold standard for the reduction of upper facial and the improvement of some lower facial lines.

line (dermal) fillers for the face

Over the last ten years in Europe, a wide variety of dermal fillers has been developed, some of which are highly successful, while others are as yet unproven and can be unsafe.

A dermal filler is a substance that is injected beneath lines in the skin, around the mouth, for example, between the nose and lips (nasolabial folds) or into deep vertical lower forehead lines. It can also be injected into sunken acne scars. It works by filling the space in the skin that is causing a hollow or line to be noticeable.

The keys to a successful dermal filler are as follows:

- once injected it should stay in place and not spread
- it should not be of animal or human origin because of the risk of allergy or disease spread; the best fillers currently are synthetic
- it should be relatively pain-free on injection
- the benefits should last for over a year
- it should not leave unwanted lumps and bumps and the risk of later allergic reactions
- it should deliver definite yet subtle improvement.

Of the fillers currently available, those that come closest to meeting the above criteria are some of the newer, longer-lasting hyaluronic acid fillers, such as Restylane and Restylane-Perlane. In studies of over 1,500 patients using these products, I found no cases of allergic reactions. This is in marked contrast to Zyderm and Zyplast which use animal or human collagen and have been shown to be much more allergenic, causing painful and unsightly reactions.

Restylane and Restylane-Perlane are produced by tricking bacteria into acting as miniature factories for hyaluronic acid. This is known as microbiologic engineering (i.e. synthesised) and results in a product that is free of anything that can lead to the transmission of human or animal diseases.

Restylane is used in different forms to achieve different goals. Restylane Fine is used for injections of the forehead and, if desired, around the eyes (although some people will develop temporary lumps). It is also sometimes injected on top of the thicker Restylane-Perlane to create, for example, a very defined look to the lip margin. Restylane is thicker than Restylane Fine and is used, in particular, for injection of the lips. Restylane-Perlane is thicker and longer lasting. It is especially valuable for treating nasolabial folds (between the nose and lips) and sunken scars. I also use it frequently for lips.

As with all treatments, fillers should be administered by an expert. This, in my opinion, would be a trained, specialised (UK) or board specialised (USA) dermatologist, dermatologic surgeon or plastic surgeon. Due to a relative shortage of dermatologists in the UK, however, others have jumped into the arena who have not undergone the appropriate training. These include nurses, general practitioners and, even more worryingly, non-medically trained and non-medically supervised beauty therapists and aestheticians. Finding the right practitioner for your chosen treatment will be covered in more detail in the Appendix, but for now, remember the guidelines on page 48, always ask for credentials, and view all advertising for cosmetic treatments with suspicion.

Before

Injections can be made painless or relatively pain-free by a combination of local anaesthetic creams under plastic tape to increase their absorption and injections of local anaesthetic into the area just before the filler is injected.

Temporary fillers:
what they can and cannot do

Can help:

- lines in the forehead and the eye area (Restylane Fine)
- to create a defined look to the lip margin (Restylane Fine + Restylane)
- nasolabial folds (Restylane-Perlane)
- sunken scars (Restylane-Perlane)

Cannot help:

- lines caused by muscle action such as crow's feet
- very deep lines from sagging skin
- eye lines from eye bags
- neck lines

Note: Restylane and Restylane-Perlane can also be used either before or during a course of NewFill (see page 83) for more immediate results.

During

Once the area is numbed the Restylane injection should be almost painless. A fine needle is inserted just under the skin and the filler injected as the needle is slowly withdrawn.

Sometimes the lips may be tender and may feel larger than they actually are due to the effects of the anaesthetic.

Length of procedure: 30–45 minutes including the local anaesthetic.

After

You should feel fine immediately after treatment and may go straight back to work. You may experience swelling for up to three or four days with lip injections, or two days with nasolabial lines. Bruising may occur, possibly

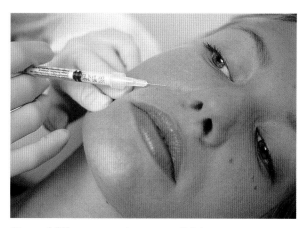

Dermal fillers can restore a youthful firmness to your lower face.

lasting up to seven days. Swelling or bruising can be concealed using a combination of green and flesh-coloured camouflage makeup which may be applied immediately after the injections if desired.

Restylane treatment aftercare

When Restylane is injected into the skin, there will be some temporary swelling and mild reddening. This is partly attributable to the filler's hyaluronic acid content which acts as a humectant (i.e. attracts water), hence the swelling. Certain people (skin phototypes 1 and 2, see page 28) will also react to the friction of the injections with mild redness which disappears, again, within a couple of days. Any swelling can be reduced with ice soaks (soak a flannel in iced water and apply to the area in question, over a ten-minute period, every four hours). Sleeping with extra pillows at night can help. Arnica tablets or cream may also help bruising, although this is not a proven treatment.

How long can the benefits of Restylane and Restylane-Perlane be expected to last?

On average the benefits may be expected to last as follows:

For lip enhancement:

Restylane	3–4 months
Restylane-Perlane	6–9 months (but can be 1 year)

For nasolabial folds or scars:

Restylane-Perlane:	12–18 months (but can be over 2 years)

For upper facial lines:

Restylane Fine	2–3 months

Possible complications

Besides the temporary swelling, redness and bruising, the only other problem that can present with Restylane and Restylane-Perlane is a temporary lumpiness, which may occur as a result of poor injection techniques, again highlighting the need for being treated by an expert. I have stopped using some of the other hyaluronic acid fillers (e.g. Hylaform) because of a higher risk of allergic reaction, which can cause painful red lumps lasting for several months. Our recent research into Restylane and Restylane-Perlane showed no allergic lumps in over 1,500 treatments. There should be no other health concerns regarding the use of Restylane and Restylane-Perlane because they are synthetic.

An exciting new development in Canada and Europe in 2004 was the new filler/implant Restylane SubQ. This is much thicker and hence longer lasting, but it requires specialist training for safe injection. It is planned to enhance cheeks, fill deep hollows and improve chins.

There are also new types of hyaluronic acid filler, but as they do not have enough research behind them, I therefore cannot recommend them.

Permanent fillers

Permanent fillers available in Europe include Artecol, Artefil, Dermalive and Bioplastique. They consist of a mixture, often of collagen or hyaluronic acid, which carries very small particles or beads into the skin through an injection. Once in the skin, the beads remain there permanently, carrying with them the risk of reactions, lumps and often painful swelling. It is virtually impossible to remove these fillers without causing scarring, and if left in place they do not always blend in with future facial changes.

Another filler that has been more widely used in the USA is silicone. Some of the newer forms of silicone, injected as tiny little droplets under the skin, are said to be safe. While it is fair to say that they carry less risk of allergic reaction than other permanent fillers (see above), silicone can cause problems as the surrounding fat under the skin is lost, leaving silicone lumps that can be seen and felt. The only solution is surgical removal. I will not treat with permanent fillers for the reasons stated.

Dermal-stimulating fillers

Dermal- or skin-stimulating fillers are an exciting new development since they act not only as fillers, but also to stimulate production of the skin's own tissues to form new collagen, or filling, of its own. One such product, NewFill, is proving to be successful; I have been using it in my London practice for over two years now with very encouraging results and it has largely replaced fat injections in my clinics.

NewFill consists of a powder made from the same chemical used to make absorbable stitches, and as such, it has a long-term safety record. It was originally developed by French dermatologists to counteract the thinning of the face that occurred in some AIDS patients being treated with new drugs. This aroused the interest of some dermatologists who were seeking to improve deep facial folds and creases. My own preference is to use NewFill for patients with very deep lines and deep scars.

It has just been approved in the USA for AIDS-related facial thinning and has been recently purchased by an American company. It is hoped that they will be developing the use of NewFill worldwide. It will be known as Sculptra.

Because NewFill is diluted with quite large volumes of fluid, the first impression immediately after injection is that the lines or scars in question have gone. However some of that fluid is then absorbed and the lines or scars will once again become partially visible. NewFill is therefore re-injected a total of three to four times over approximately a four-month period (i.e. at three- to six-week intervals). Following each injection, the skin is stimulated to produce more and more of its own collagen and subcutaneous tissue, which then gradually fills the lines or scars.

Before, during and after treatment with NewFill

Before

As well as using local anaesthetic creams, local anaesthetic is mixed with NewFill to reduce pain.

During

The NewFill is injected into the deeper dermis or subcutaneous layer. A minimal pinprick sensation is felt during the treatment.

Length of procedure: 30–60 minutes including numbing the skin with local anaesthetic.

After

Some bruising and swelling will be apparent and possibly some temporary lumps. You can return to work after treatment and camouflage makeup may be applied.

NewFill treatment aftercare

No special aftercare is needed with NewFill.

Possible complications

One of the original problems with NewFill was that some physicians were injecting it too superficially and in too concentrated a form. This led to some lumps that went away in time. Used in a more dilute form and injected slightly deeper, however, NewFill does not present any such problems, but it is probably best avoided in the lips.

NewFill:
what it can and cannot do   * * *   * * *

Can help:

- deep folds, lines and creases
- deep scars
- increasing prominence of cheekbone area.

Cannot help:

- severely sagging skin
- sunspots
- drooping eyelids

Note: in the future NewFill may be used to inject the neck, chest (décolletage) and the back of the hands, once further research into these areas has been carried out.

Other fillers – your own fat

Another process that has become popular in the last decade is that of injecting a patient's own fat into deep facial lines and scars. The fat is usually obtained from the lower stomach or thighs, following an injection of dilute local anaesthesia. It is then processed using a variety of techniques, collectively known as a fat transfer procedure.

My own preference is to do as little as possible with the fat before re-injecting to avoid incurring any damage to it. I will generally harvest enough fat for a year's worth of injections and freeze it. The fat is then re-injected, usually every six to eight weeks, on at least four or five occasions over the course of a year. There is evidence to suggest that in some people the fat lasts for over a year and may also stimulate the growth of new fat and subcutaneous tissues. In others it may only last a few months.

Fat harvesting should always be carried out by a specialist surgeon or physician and in sterile conditions. Very occasionally, small particles of fat may enter a blood vessel and this can lead to an ulcer in the skin that may heal with some scarring.

In general I would use fat injections for the same situations as NewFill (see above); some people prefer to avoid using any foreign material in their skin and for them their own fat is a useful filler.

Before, during and after a fat transfer procedure

Before
Do not take any blood-thinning medication, aspirin or arthritis medicine as this may cause an increased risk of bruising.

During
You will have a very dilute solution of anaesthetic run under your skin with a fine needle.

Length of procedure: 60 minutes for fat harvesting, 15–30 for fat injections.

After
You may be swollen and bruised where the fat is injected. With small amounts of fat injection, you can go back to work.

> ∗ **WARNING!** ∗
>
> Fat should not be injected into the forehead as it can enter veins and may cause blindness if particles reach the blood vessels in the eyes. The injections may also damage facial nerves.

new implants for deeper lines and thin lips

A new development in this area is an implant known as UltraSoft, which is a very soft and flexible type of tubular Gore-Tex. Gore-Tex has been used in the body for well over 30 years to repair blood vessels, stomach walls and other organs. It is known to be safe and does not cause allergic reactions.

One of the benefits of treatment with UltraSoft is that the implants can be removed if the person's face changes (for example, if it becomes thinner so that the implant shows through) or, in very rare cases if the implant moves (for example, if the face is hit in an accident). One patient of mine was playing golf and was hit on the side of her face with a golf ball. I removed the displaced UltraSoft and substituted it later with another UltraSoft implant.

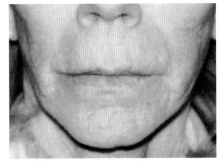

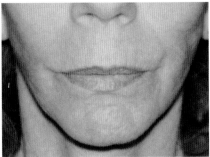

Subtle filling with lip implants leads to a more balanced, sensuous mouth.

As with all treatments, UltraSoft needs to be implanted by a dermatologic surgeon or plastic surgeon who has been specially trained in its use.

UltraSoft implants: what they can and cannot do

* * *

* * *

Can help:

- to achieve subtle but permanent enlargement of very thin lips
- to fill deep nasolabial folds

Cannot help:

- scars
- lines on the cheeks
- forehead lines

liposuction of the face, chin and neck

This procedure has been greatly improved over the last 15 years by dermatologic surgeons in the USA, pioneered by Dr Jeffery Klein of southern California who has been responsible for many of the refinements made to liposuction techniques. These include 'tumescent local anaesthesia liposuction'. 'Tumescent' refers to the large volumes of very dilute anaesthesia that are injected through tiny tubes or cannulas into the fat layer below the skin from which the patient is to have fat removed. The technique has proved to be highly successful and, more importantly, very safe (as opposed to liposuction under general anaesthesia following which several cases of death or serious illness have been reported both in Europe and in the USA). It is practised now by dermatologic surgeons and some plastic surgeons who have been trained in its use.

However, liposuction of the face and neck is not suitable for everybody. As with all procedures, an evaluation of the patient must be undertaken by the dermatologic surgeon or plastic surgeon. The ideal patient for this procedure on the neck is someone who has an accumulation of fat pads under the chin, causing the jaw line to disappear. It would not be an appropriate procedure, though, for someone with very loose skin as this will not tighten back after liposuction.

Fat that has collected on the lower face (i.e. the jaw line or 'jowls') can also benefit from liposuction. However, this is often accompanied by a hollowing of the cheeks, and if the former is addressed without tackling the latter, the face can end up looking more drawn and aged. The hollowing should therefore be dealt with separately by harvesting fat from another part of the body (see page 85) and injecting it into the cheeks, while the jowl problem is solved with liposuction.

For very lax, loose, aged and sun-damaged skin referral to a plastic surgeon will be required. They will usually perform a face and neck lift – a more serious surgical procedure with general anaesthesia and recovery time lasting up to several weeks.

Before, during and after treatment with liposuction

Before

You will be given an antibiotic to start a day before treatment. Also all medication that might increase the risk of bruising (e.g. aspirin and arthritis medications) should be stopped. Blood pressure and heart rate readings will be taken before the procedure.

Liposuction of the face, chin and neck: what it can and cannot do

* * *   * * *

Can help:

- to remove fat pads from under the chin ('double' or 'triple chin') and fat that has collected around the jowls

Cannot help:

- very lax or excess skin, as this skin will not tighten back after treatment
- sun-damaged skin

During

Very dilute local anaesthesia is infused (injected) through tiny cannulas into the relevant fatty area/s. No sedation is required and after the anaesthesia takes effect, the fat is removed through suction apparatus, via the cannulas. There should be no pain or discomfort during or after liposuction. Some patients will have tiny stitches and these will need to be removed between five and seven days after the procedure.

Length of procedure: 60–90 minutes plus removal of stitches later.

After

It is possible to go about your normal daily activities without any restriction. There will be some bruising in the neck, but you can camouflage this with makeup or wear high-necked shirts until the bruising has gone.

Liposuction aftercare

I usually supply a special neck support garment that can be taken off easily when you want to go out. This tends to speed the tightening of the neck.

Possible complications

It can sometimes be difficult to judge exactly how much fat to remove, so fat can be left in some areas, while in others too much may be inadvertently removed, which can lead to hollowing. This can usually be corrected, however, using fat transfer (see page 85). Another very rare but possible complication is that of nerve damage leading to numbness, tingling or muscle weakness of the lower face.

Infection is still a remote possibility. This would show as swelling, pain and redness under the skin and a prolonged course of antibiotics may be required. You should only have liposuction treatment if you are completely healthy at the outset.

facial hair and its removal

The presence of facial hair is often undesirable for women, and can make them feel uncomfortable and unfeminine, impacting on their self-esteem. This can rarely lead to profound psychological and emotional problems, which have to be addressed by the dermatologist, who may then organise referrals for psychotherapy or counselling.

Some women, particularly those from Middle Eastern and Mediterranean countries, have greater hair density on their face and body than do women with lighter skin types, from, for example, northern Europe.

In some cases, especially in younger women, there is a medical reason for facial hair growth and it is important for the dermatologist to rule out any such cause. One example would be an excess of male hormones produced by the ovaries and adrenal glands, or it can be part of a combination of problems that includes facial acne plus cysts on the ovaries, which is known as polycystic ovarian syndrome. If you have acne that extends into your 20s or 30s, together with excess hair, your dermatologist may arrange for you to undergo blood and ovary-scanning investigations.

Very occasionally pregnant women may produce excessive facial hair growth, usually accompanied by a heavy growth of scalp hair. Some medications, such as cortisone or some blood pressure medications, can also result in hair growth.

However, in most cases facial hair growth occurs in women without any obvious underlying medical cause, but it is still felt by them to be a sign of ageing. In later life, women do undergo changes in facial hair growth, particularly around the time of the menopause, when the hair may become coarser and darker or whiter.

It should come as no surprise, therefore, that facial hair removal is one of the procedures I find most often requested by women.

Electrolysis

First used in 1875, electrolysis involves an electric current, which is passed through a fine wire needle introduced into the area around the hair, which damages the hair root, causing the hair to be destroyed. The procedure is very effective if you have a small number of coarse facial hairs and may, in fact, be the only viable option for coarse white hairs. However, it does become impractical in cases of multiple hair growth, for example on the lower face, and can occasionally, if used too frequently, cause scarring. Research is currently under way into newer laser machines, which may reduce white or grey hair.

Before, during and after treatment with electrolysis

Before
Avoid waxing, plucking or shaving – the practitioner has to be able to see your hair.

During
Local anaesthetic creams may be applied as this can be a painful procedure. A tiny needle is inserted along the hair and an electric current released, killing the follicle.

Length of procedure: depends on the extent of the area to be treated but should range from 30 minutes for the upper lip to an hour for larger areas. It is difficult to tolerate this treatment for longer than 1 hour because of the discomfort.

After
There will be some redness and occasionally swelling if a large area has been treated. You can apply makeup immediately and go straight back to work if desired.

Electrolysis treatment aftercare
No special aftercare is needed.

Possible complications
There can be some scabbing or crusting (i.e. infection) following the procedure. If performed too frequently in an area such as the upper lip, it can lead to small ice-pick scars and loss of pigment.

Laser hair removal
For people with more extensive hair growth, laser hair removal has become the treatment of choice. Some modern lasers are highly effective at reducing hair that has some pigment, although very blond, white, grey and, in some cases, red hair respond poorly. Some recent advances in laser and light technology may succeed with white and grey hair.

For white or very fine grey hair, waxing, shaving or electrolysis are viable options, followed by the use of Vaniqua cream, developed to reduce the regrowth of hair following removal for up to several weeks. This cream is available on prescription.

The potential for laser hair removal was originally discovered by accident when it was noted during a tattoo removal procedure that the Ruby laser also reduced hair growth. Today, there are over 25 different laser or light systems that claim to be effective for laser hair removal. Consult an expert to help you with choices and decisions.

Before, during and after laser hair removal treatment

Before
Minimise your sun exposure and tanning (this includes sunless tans).

During
Skin will be cooled with the modern laser, which will reduce pain. Local anaesthetic cream may also be applied to tender skin areas. You will feel a mild 'zapping' sensation like that of a rubber band against the skin when the laser light is released.

Length of procedure: 10–60 minutes, depending on the area being treated (10 minutes for the upper lip and chin and up to 60 minutes for the back or thighs).

* * * **Laser hair removal: the myths and the facts** * * *

Myth Laser hair removal is permanent.

Fact It is not permanent but it can achieve long-term reduction in growth, and the subsequent regrowth is lighter and less noticeable.

Myth One treatment will do the job.

Fact Several treatments are required – possibly between three and six depending on hair colour and texture – for maximum benefit.

Myth You cannot go out in the sun after treatment.

Fact You can go out in the sun, but use a broad-spectrum sunscreen to reduce tanning. If you are tanned after a vacation, your laser dermatologist will often advise to delay further treatment until the tan has reduced.

After

You can go straight back to work after treatment. Again, minimise your sun exposure throughout the course of treatment and for four weeks after it has finished. Use a broad-spectrum sunscreen and apply makeup if desired.

Laser hair removal treatment aftercare

Continue to use sunscreens and avoid getting tanned if you are having a course of several laser treatments.

Possible complications

Permanent pigment loss can occur in people with darker skin (phototypes 3–6, see pages 28–29) if the wrong laser or the wrong energy level is used. Also, if skin is overcooled during treatment abnormal pigmentation can result. For safest results, laser hair removal should be carried out by, or under the direct guidance of a dermatology specialist trained in laser therapy.

Pulsed light systems for hair removal

Some of the pulsed light systems (see pages 63–64) can be used for hair removal. In general, more treatments would be required than with lasers and they also tend to take longer to show improvements; however, they can be very successful. Greater care is needed again with these long-pulsed light systems in people with darker skin (phototypes 3–6, see pages 28–29).

For details of treatment, see laser hair removal, above.

Combined medical and laser hair removal

Some people benefit from a combination approach of lasers plus prescription medical treatments. Women whose excess hair growth stems from a hormonal problem may be treated with an oral contraceptive – Dianette (not approved in the USA) and Yasmin, which blocks the hormones' effects on the hair follicles. Another option is Spironolactone, a water pill which has been found to have weak Dianette-like properties. However, it is essential to consult a dermatologist regarding these drugs. In the UK dermatologists are also fully trained general physicians, who will have had training in diseases of internal organs, including hormone problems) and are, as such, qualified to deal with such oral medication. Elsewhere you may be referred to a hormone specialist (endocrinologist) for help.

cosmetic surgery: a brief overview

Cosmetic surgery is a vast field in its own right and, as such, it really falls beyond the scope of this book. However, it is useful to know a little bit about it in order to put it into some sort of context as regards options for facial rejuvenation as a whole.

Plastic surgery was developed in both the United States and Europe from early in the twentieth century. Initially, it was practised for reconstructive needs, to correct deformities in both children and adults, whether congenital (such as cleft palate and cleft lip), or trauma-induced, following accidents or injury. Injuries sustained in the Second World War, in particular, led to many advances in reconstructive surgery. From plastic and reconstructive surgery, the overlapping speciality of aesthetic or cosmetic surgery has evolved, to the extent that in the first part of this century there were probably over 3 million cosmetic surgical procedures in the USA and over 60,000 in the United Kingdom per year.

Cosmetic surgery, performed by a skilled surgeon, can be very successful, either on its own or as part of a combined facial rejuvenation programme, in helping to improve the following:

- face sagging
- neck sagging or ageing
- drooping brow
- upper eyelid drooping
- 'bags' under the eyes
- nose shape

It can also help to improve some ageing of the body (breasts can be lifted, reduced or enlarged, post-pregnancy stretched abdomens and stomach walls can be tightened).

As with all forms of treatment, and as I have stressed throughout the book, it is essential to be well informed and to consult only practitioners who have the appropriate credentials (see Appendix, pages 144–153, for more detailed advice). Cosmetic surgery does require general anaesthesia (with its associated risks) as well as time out for recovery and some scars may be visible.

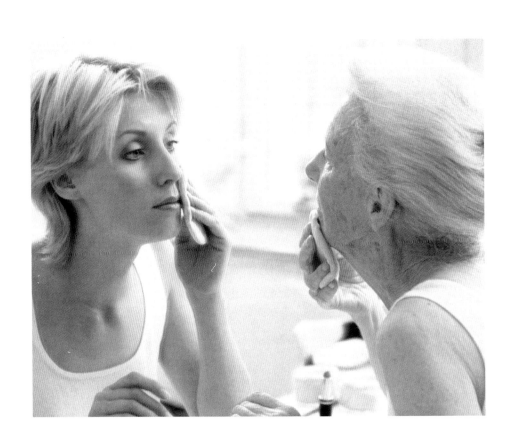

chapter four

creams, topical potions and sunscreens

Open any glossy beauty or fashion magazine and you will be bombarded with advertising from cosmetic companies who would have us all believe that their products fall little short of the 'fountain of youth'. While there is real evidence to support the success of some of the prescription retinoid creams (Retin-A, Tazarotene – see pages 107–110), the myths abound regarding the rejuvenating properties of many cosmetic creams, serums and lotions. As we have seen in earlier chapters, the ageing face is characterised by a number of different features including fine wrinkles, deeper wrinkles, blotchy pigmentations, spider veins, a rough texture, often an unhealthy or sallow colour but these, despite manufacturers' claims, cannot be improved by creams and lotions alone, and especially not in a few days.

Myth Botulinum toxin (Botox) and/or collagen in a cream can work wonders.

Fact These molecules are too large to penetrate the skin and cannot therefore work in a cream.

Myth Wrinkle-decreasing and nightly renewal creams are effective skin rejuvenators.

Fact If they produce any improvement, this is likely to be the result of temporary skin hydration and at best will only provide a slight benefit beyond that of moisturisation. This can be helpful if you are prone to dry skin.

Myth Oxygen in a cream is essential for young skin.

Fact Creams probably do not deliver oxygen to the skin but, even if they do, your skin should already get plenty from your blood unless you are a heavy smoker.

So how can you steer clear of becoming victims of advertising hype? How is it possible to sort out what is effective from what is not? And how do you avoid spending large sums of money on expensive topical creams that really have no advantage over reliable, inexpensive creams? The answer is to obtain your information from an impartial dermatologist (some physicians, surgeons and scientists may have vested interests in particular products and may endorse them because of this) and to bear in mind that more expensive does not necessarily mean more effective.

Consider the following:

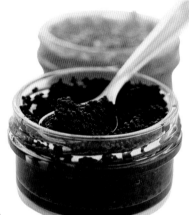

- *A cream developed by a NASA scientist based on marine ingredients:* this claims to have special properties because of its marine algae content. However there is little or no scientific proof that this concept has any special benefits in human skin, although it is probably a good moisturiser.

- *An expensive cream containing caviar eggs:* it may be an effective moisturiser, but how does it compare with less expensive, reliable creams? It may be better to eat the caviar as it should have a high concentration of omega-3 fatty acids which may help your heart!

Eat caviar, don't apply it.

- *A skin-care programme promoted by a dermatologist that recommends that eating large quantities of salmon is good for the skin:* there is scientific data to support the fact that a diet that is high in oily fish seems to reduce the risk of heart disease but is there any convincing data to suggest that it helps to protect against skin ageing? I am unaware of any credible scientific evidence to support the idea that eating salmon or herring or tuna (even the deliciously fatty toro for sushi fans) is beneficial to the skin, although it is good for the heart. The antioxidant, anti-ageing, anti-inflammatory benefits of this diet on the skin have yet to be scientifically proven. Also beware that oily fish may contain high levels of toxins, depending on where they are farmed or fished.

A great variety of creams can be found containing just about anything from fish egg extracts to plant ingredients and marine algae, making highly exaggerated claims and costing a fortune to buy. While they may not actually harm you, their benefits will certainly not justify their cost. In contrast, studies have been carried out using some types of aloe vera which do have a limited ability to reduce inflammation in the skin and it is possible to buy inexpensive aloe vera creams. However, the benefits of aloe vera are far fewer than those of prescription creams.

Vaseline Intensive Care is an excellent example of an all-over-body lotion that contains a multiple vitamin complex just like that hyped in some of the very expensive creams, but one that is easily found at the local pharmacy and at a fraction of the cost. Other large companies such as Unilever, Proctor & Gamble, L'Oréal and Johnson & Johnson all manufacture products that are extremely well formulated and thoroughly tested. They give the skin a smooth and healthy appearance, are cosmetically sound, and they don't break the bank either. It is important to realise, however, that non-prescription cosmetic creams that are bought 'over the counter' will only offer at best a slight benefit with regard to facial ageing. Such benefit will not be nearly as great or as long term as it would be in the case of a prescription cream such as Retin-A or Tazarotene.

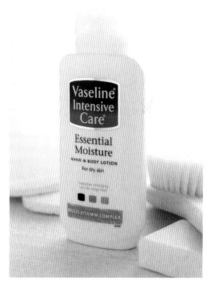

The cost of a product is not related to its effectiveness.

What to look for in the 'active' ingredients of creams:

- Moisturisation – from humectants such as glycerine or sodium hyduronate

- Antioxidant mixtures, e.g. vitamin E (tocopherols), vitamin C (ascorbic acid, ascorbyl palmitate)

- Low levels of retinoids such as retinol, retinaldehyde and vitamin A

cosmeceuticals

Cosmeceuticals are essentially cosmetics, but have been shown in some trials and also in some cell culture studies to demonstrate potential benefits for skin rejuvenation. They are called cosmeceuticals because even though they are cosmetics they do show some mild activity similar to that of a pharmaceutical cream so, Cosmetic + Pharmaceutical = Cosmeceutical. The 'father' of skin ageing research and Retin-A, Dr Albert Kligman of the University of Pennsylvania, coined this term about 20 years ago. The marketing claims for cosmeceuticals are carefully designed to avoid regulation by the licensing authorities (for example, the Medical Control Agency in the UK, European Commission on Cosmetics, the Food and Drug Administration – FDA – in the USA). They are scientifically designed topical products, they have appropriate pleasing characteristics (e.g. neither too dry nor too greasy) and they meet chemical, pharmaceutical and medical standards but their manufacturers have to be very careful not to make claims that would make them pharmaceuticals, i.e. they are not allowed to say that they change the structure and function of the skin. If the products were classed as pharmaceutical prescription creams, they would then be required to undergo extensive and expensive research and testing.

However, there are many ingredients in cosmeceuticals that are at best confusing for shoppers and despite the new rules relating to the labelling of all important ingredients, it is very difficult for even the informed consumer to be aware of what the different substances do, are supposed to do, or in many instances fail to do. So let's now take a look at just what's on the cosmeceutical menu.

* * *   **Examples of cosmeceuticals**   * * *

- Creams containing 5–10 per cent glycolic acid

- 'Rejuvenating' creams containing retinol or retinaldehyde e.g. Roc Retinol products

- 'Rejuvenating' creams containing vitamin C ingredients that probably increase collagen production, e.g. SkinCeuticals C

Vitamin and vitamin-like cosmeceutical ingredients

While the value of oral supplementation with vitamins at the recommended daily amounts is not disputed for the maintenance of general health, the benefits of larger doses for the correction of certain health disorders has been seriously challenged of late in many scientific publications. Similarly, the usefulness of some non-prescription topical vitamin applications remains controversial. Some products may offer a modest benefit but will not be nearly as effective as the prescription products. For example, a cosmetic product containing small amounts of vitamin A or retinol cannot hope to compare with prescription strengths of vitamin A (such as Retin-A or Tazarotene, see pages 107–110) in terms of improving ageing skin.

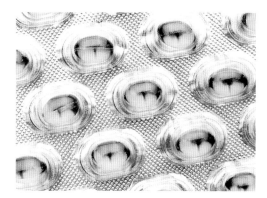

Oral vitamin supplements can be highly effective in maintaining good health, but only a few, such as vitamins A and C, have proven topical benefits.

Vitamin A

This is essential for the maintenance of normal human skin as well as for general health. Vitamin A is one of a family of natural and synthetic products that are incorporated into both prescription and non-prescription anti-ageing creams known as retinoids. I have been studying the effects of retinoids on the skin for over 25 years and the bottom line seems to be that some of these agents are highly effective at skin rejuvenation, for example Retin-A and Tazarotene gels and creams. These have to be obtained from a physician, preferably your dermatologist, with instructions on how to use them. Other products that contain agents such as retinyl palmitate, retinaldehyde and retinol can be shown to have milder effects on skin rejuvenation.

It is also likely that small amounts of naturally occurring vitamin A, such as retinyl palmitate and retinol, act as antioxidants (see page 101) but whether or not these amounts are enough to have any observable long-term benefits on the skin has yet to be proven.

Vitamin C

There is a great deal of hype and misinformation about vitamin C. It is known to act both as an antioxidant, scavenging and quenching free radicals (chemicals formed in the cells of the body in response to chemical or sunlight damage) and also as a very important factor in the production of collagen structures. We know, for example, that vitamin C taken orally is essential for wound healing and also that in scurvy (extreme vitamin C deficiency) sailors developed difficulty in healing skin wounds. Of course this is an extreme condition to which most people today are not exposed. Captain James Cook, the explorer, is credited with having fed his crew vegetables and fruit such as cabbages and limes, with a high content of vitamin C, in order to prevent scurvy. This gave the British Navy advantages over the French and Spanish, although whether the British sailors had younger-looking skin was never recorded!

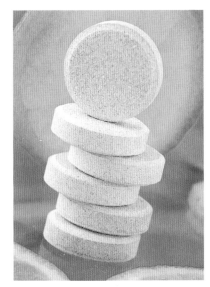

Creams containing vitamin C may create new collagen and reduce sunburn.

Correctly formulated, some of the vitamin C-containing creams are highly effective in quenching free radicals and also in reducing some of the immediate effects of sunlight (sunburn, for example) and the number of damaged cells produced by sunlight. However, while it is possible that they may have some mild sun protection properties, it is unknown whether prolonged use of vitamin C-containing creams can result in skin rejuvenation and repair, and generally speaking they are extremely varied in their benefits. Some research studies in animals suggest a reduction in the risk of skin cancer when using vitamin C-, vitamin E- and selenium-containing creams or oral solutions but there is no good evidence to show that this is the case in humans. Mice and men are quite different experimentally!

One of the problems with topical vitamin C preparations is that they are not always stable, meaning that in many instances the vitamin C does not penetrate the skin as the active intact substance. It is therefore essential to know that the cream in question does actually deliver the vitamin C to the skin, which is something you should check with your dermatologist.

If you *are* going to use a vitamin C preparation, which ones actually work? The SkinCeuticals range, formulated by a dermatologist in the USA, contains a 10 per cent concentration (quite a large proportion) of ascorbic acid (the chemical name for a stable vitamin C) and appears to reduce the immediate effects of sunlight (sunburn) as well as stimulate collagen-forming chemicals, at least experimentally. We do not as yet have proof that it actually forms enough collagen to reduce wrinkles, but given the experimental studies it is likely that it has a good chance to do so. Look for the words 'stabilised vitamin C' on product labels. Certain products have been tested for their ability to reduce sunlight-induced skin damage and these tend to be the more thoroughly researched products. I generally advise people to use vitamin C-containing creams if they have mild existing sun damage and want to minimise the risk of incurring new sun damage. Also some people can tolerate vitamin C-containing creams but not Retin-A.

Coenzyme Q10

Coenzyme Q10, another vitamin-like substance, is thought to have excellent antioxidant free radical-quenching properties. Because of this, it tends to be added to skin treatment creams such as moisturisers, especially those that make claims of rejuvenation. There is some evidence to suggest that coenzyme Q10 in products such as Eucerin or Nivea can help in skin protection.

Vitamin E

Vitamin E is also known as tocopherol or tocopherol acetate. Again, as with the above vitamins, it is thought to be an important antioxidant which has been shown in studies to reduce sunburn and skin cancer in animals exposed to artificial sunlight. The

* * * **Antioxidants** * * *

While a mixture of pomegranates, grapes and citrus fruits may sound like a rather exotic fruit salad, there is new research to suggest that it may act as a powerful weapon against skin cancer. Experiments, which have thus far been carried out on mice, have shown that these fruits have high levels of antioxidant activity. Should these exciting results be backed up by studies on humans, it may be that skin cancer-fighting creams and sunscreens containing extracts of these fruits could be coming to our pharmacies in the not-too-distant future.

problem is that this has not been shown to be the case in human skin. It has also been proposed that vitamin E can reduce heart disease. Conversely, the popular conception that vitamin E cream helps skin wounds to heal better and faster has not been proven. The most active type of vitamin E is alpha tocopherol.

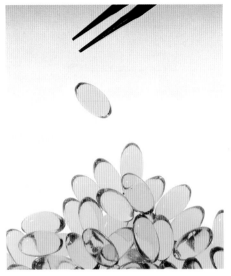

Oral vitamin E supplements can reduce the blood-clotting ability which means that the vitamin E must be stopped several days before any sort of surgery to reduce the risks of bruising. (This is also true of cosmetic procedures involving injections, such as Botox and skin fillers.)

Is topical vitamin E an effective antioxidant and protection for human skin? We do not know for sure, but one study suggested that in laboratory tests on the skin, alpha tocopherol is a very effective antioxidant.

Alphalipoic acid

Oral vitamin C is being researched for heart disease and prostrate cancer prevention; in a cream, it may reduce skin ageing and skin cancers.

This is a free radical-quenching fatty acid that has been suggested to have superior ability in protecting and rejuvenating the skin. Considerable publicity associated with this ingredient has been generated by an American dermatologist, who also advocates a diet high in salmon as a skin rejuvenator. While I would consider the possibility that alphalipoic acid can act as a free radical scavenger (protector) in the skin, I feel that more scientific evidence is required to support its value as a rejuvenator as compared with that of other ingredients. In fact, a scientific presentation at the 2004 American Academy of Dermatology showed that in several research tests alphalipoic acid was a less potent antioxidant than others including tocophorol.

Superoxide dismutase (SOD) – a powerful antioxidant

This has been shown to be a highly effective antioxidant in test tube and animal studies and may be helpful in protecting the skin against free radical damage. Again, it is not known for certain just how useful it is clinically in terms of human skin. More studies are required to determine its long-term benefits but it is being used in some creams, is unlikely to be harmful and may prove to be a good skin-protecting agent.

Myth Words or phrases such as 'natural', 'botanical' and 'plant-derived' indicate a safer, more effective product.

Fact Some of the most toxic and allergenic substances known to man are derived from plants, so do not assume that a 'natural' product is going to be superior to a synthetic one. Some botanicals are effective for anti-inflammatory purposes, e.g. chamomile and pomegranate extract. Others are mild skin lighteners, e.g. liquorice extract.

botanical ingredients

Creams can incorporate a whole range of botanical ingredients, some of which may not necessarily be effective but are used because it is then permissible to say that the product in question is a botanical – a natural cream containing natural plant extracts and botanical ingredients, which may be attractive to the consumer. A variety of botanicals is used, including pomegranate extract, grapefruit extract, calendula, aloe vera and liquorice extract.

Flavenoids such as green tea extract and ginkgo biloba have been shown to have effective anti-free radical, anti-damaging properties in some cell culture systems and animal studies. However, there has been little in the way of controlled scientific studies into their value in skin creams in humans and it does, I think, require a big leap of faith to take something that apparently works in the test tube, add it to a cream, and expect it to have the same benefits. Having said that, most botanical products are probably harmless. They may, at worst, be unhelpful, and at best, offer slight benefits with regard to reducing inflammation from the harmful effects of ultraviolet light. Some future developments in green tea and gingko biloba may lead to skin creams that have sun protection and age-reversal ability. Certainly, some green tea extracts have been shown to be capable of reducing ultraviolet-induced (artificial sunlight) skin swelling in some animal studies.

Echinacea is derived from flowers originating in North America used by native Americans as a skin preparation. It is a common botanical ingredient and is thought to act as both an anti-inflammatory and moisturiser, reducing irritancy in the skin.

Aloe vera has also been used for many years in a variety of creams and gels. It is an important extract of the aloe plant and offers a variety of different benefits. Studies have confirmed that it can help to reduce inflammation and improve wound healing. In order for it to provide beneficial moisturising effects on the skin, aloe vera must be present at a concentration of 10 per cent, below which it is unlikely to be effective. Whether or not this agent has any anti-skin-ageing benefits is not known at this time but, again, its anti-inflammatory properties make it a useful and effective ingredient in general skin maintenance.

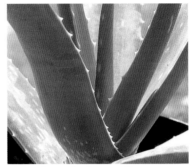

Some botanical ingredients may help to improve skin quality.

moisturising ingredients

Moisturising ingredients work by a variety of different mechanisms in the skin.

One way is to operate as a moisture trap. An example of this would be Vaseline or Petrolatum, which enter the upper outer layers of the stratum corneum (see page 12) preventing increased water loss. Then, with the help of this protective barrier, the skin is able to reduce water loss. There is a possibility that Petrolatum can cause

Myth Cosmeceuticals and non-prescription creams offer highly effective skin rejuvenation properties.

Fact They may be beneficial in moisturising terms, but have minimal skin rejuvenation powers.

Myth The more a cream costs, the better it is.

Fact There is absolutely no need to spend large sums of money on this type of cream. Vaseline Intensive Care moisturiser for dry skin, for example, contains added multiple vitamins (retinyl palmitate, tocopherol acetate, panthenol and sodium PCA, as well as excellent humectants such as glycerine and urea) and retails in the UK at a fraction of the cost of other products that may boast all sorts of rare and expensive ingredients but are not scientifically proven and simply do not make the grade. A dermatologist should be able to help you through the cosmeceutical maze.

acne and my feeling is that it is often the frequency of the application and the extent of rubbing of the skin with Petrolatum that is likely to cause acne, but it is probably best to avoid using it on the face (see also page 106). Acne may also be more likely to occur if Petrolatum is applied and then covered under a headband or a cap.

Moisturisers can also function as humectants, i.e. by actually attracting water into the stratum corneum to hydrate the skin. Examples of this are glycerine and sodium hyaluronate, both of which are excellent moisturising ingredients.

There are, in addition, 'natural' moisturising factors. These contain a mixture of different amino acids and salts designed to mimic the natural composition of the stratum corneum. If the skin is lacking in natural moisturisers, it will certainly become cracked and dry, so these, or a chemical called sodium PCA, may be added to some products to prevent this from happening.

Urea is a chemical moisturising ingredient that comes with its own benefits and drawbacks. On the positive side, it helps to create a more even stratum corneum by smoothing out the skin's surface. However, on the downside, being an acid means that urea can both sting and irritate and also smell rather unpleasant.

Fruit acids

Fruit acids (or alpha-hydroxy acids – AHAs – which include glycolic acid, lactic acid, citric acid, mandelic acid and tartaric acid) are also known as hydroxyl acids and have been known since ancient times to be beneficial in improving the smoothness and general feel of the skin. The ancient Egyptians would collect grapeseed remains containing tartaric acid from the bottom of their wine-fermenting vessels and apply them to their skin to make it smooth and glowing.

In modern times, the most commonly used fruit acid is glycolic acid. In the USA it is allowed in non-prescription creams at up to 5 per cent concentrations and while higher concentrations are available, they need to be dispensed by a physician. These regulations have not been adopted in Europe or elsewhere although perhaps they ought to be, as such creams can cause redness or irritation in people with problems such as sensitive skin or eczema, for example. In general, however, glycolic acid-containing lotions or creams will help to promote a smoother, healthier-looking skin.

Panthenol

Panthenol, or vitamin B5, is used in a variety of skin and hair products including shampoos, conditioners and moisturisers. It is very useful as a humectant, attracting moisture into hair and skin. It smooths the surface of skin and hair and has also been shown to help in wound healing. It is sometimes used in a form known as calcium pantothenate (e.g. in Neutrogena Healthy Defence moisturiser).

Niacinamide (Nicotinamide) – a new use for an old chemical

This is a chemical that has been shown to have some interesting and important actions on the skin. One of these is to reduce redness and inflammation. In experiments on animal skin, it has been seen to reduce skin ageing that is a result of artificial sunlight as well as reducing the risk of skin cancer. It is not yet known whether this is also the case in humans, but it is nevertheless being used in 'anti-ageing' moisturisers such as Olay Total Effects Anti-ageing Complex. Another recently discovered valuable property is its ability to improve acne. In both the UK and the USA it is used in a prescription gel at a concentration of 4 per cent (Nicam gel). Whether or not it has any anti-acne potential at lower strengths (as it is found in non-prescription preparations) is not known.

Lipids

Lipids are fats that form a natural part of the skin's barrier. The most important lipids in the skin are ceremides, sphingolipids, sterols and free fatty acids. All of these are essential for the skin barrier to function. Some moisturisers contain a mixture of these skin barrier lipids or chemical variants of them, sometimes known as ceramides. Often they are combined with humectants such as glycerine to produce an effective moisturiser such as Vaseline Intensive Care.

Petrolatum (petroleum jelly)

This is used in hand and body moisturisers but should not, in my opinion, be applied to the skin on the face (although it is good for dry lips) because it can cause blackheads, whiteheads and acne in susceptible skin types. It needs to be produced by a reliable manufacturer because it can contain contaminants such as tars, which can be harmful and pose a skin cancer risk if it is used long term.

growth factors

These are 'biological cosmeceuticals/pharmaceuticals' that can be obtained from human cell lines. Some are used as 'stem cells' for treating severe disease such as cancer and leukaemia. They are sometimes also used after chemotherapy to boost the body's defences. It is not known whether they really work well in human skin to reduce ageing, however the theory is that growth factors will stimulate new collagen and elastin which will, in turn, lead to more resilient skin. These chemicals are big molecules that work in the test tube but which the skin may find difficult to absorb.

copper peptides

These have been recently introduced and have rejuvenating properties in cell culture studies – more research is needed to discover their true benefits.

topical anti-ageing prescription creams

Vitamin A is of vital importance to the normal development and maintenance of the skin and other organs, and its importance cannot be overstated. The skin needs vitamin A to control the formation of hair, nails and teeth (the teeth are derived from the skin), as well as that of normal epidermis. Vitamin A regulates the way in which the epidermis matures into the stratum corneum (see page 12).

Only the retinoid creams that contain prescription 'retinoid' substances related to vitamin A have been scientifically proven to improve skin ageing. Long-term studies of these creams have shown increased collagen formation and renewed epidermis.

The most proven prescription skin-renewing cream – Retin-A

All-trans retinoic acid, also known as Tretinoin, has been a prescription form of topical vitamin A for 45 years and is the active ingredient in Retin-A and now in other generic retinoids. Retin-A has been used since the 1960s for treating acne and therefore has a long proven history of safety. There is no evidence that it increases the risk of sunlight sensitivity in human skin, although this is one of several myths that surround Retin-A.

If it is used too frequently or at too high a strength Tretinoin (Retin-A) cream can cause problems with skin dryness, redness and flaking (tretinoin dermatitis).

However, these side effects are avoidable and some of the lower-strength creams (e.g. Retin-A 0.025 per cent) used nightly, on alternate nights or even every third night, can reverse skin ageing. The gels tend to be more drying than creams so I generally recommend creams to my patients.

Retin-A cream can be used safely on skin showing early signs of ageing and also used as part of a combination treatment with chemical peels, microdermabrasion, Botox and fillers in more severely aged skin. In some cases, I would start Retin-A cream in patients as young as 25 if they have signs of early sun-induced skin ageing.

How does Retin-A counter or reduce skin ageing?

Tretinoin (Retin-A) creams improve the outer layers of the skin by increasing the production of more normal-looking cells (in sun-damaged skin the cells become strange-looking with altered contents such as the nucleus). By increasing cell production, they shed blotchy, dark pigment from the skin and also increase collagen formation in the dermis, both directly and as a result of increased outer skin layer production. The result is a brighter, healthier-looking and more supple skin with fewer fine lines and blotchy dark patches and a more resilient feel.

* * *   Retin-A in other forms   * * *

Retin-A has been more recently formulated in ointments or 'moisturising creams' that were supposed to reduce the drying effects of Retin-A. One of these is called Retinova or Renova. One problem I have seen with this preparation is that it is too 'greasy' for some people and leads to whiteheads and acne. This problem is known as 'comedogenis' or 'acnegenesis'. It is also a problem with some of the more greasy cosmetics, makeups and sunscreens. Look for the words 'non-acnegenic' or 'non-comedogenic' on the packaging.

Other formulations enclose the Retin-A in microspheres of fat which slowly release the Retin-A into the skin. This is again in an attempt to reduce irritancy. I prefer to control irritancy by reducing the frequency of application and also by reducing the length of time that the Retin-A or Tazarotene (see page 110) actually sits on the skin before it is washed off.

Using Retin-A

People who are starting on Retin-A, in particular those who have a sensitive skin, always begin with Retin-A 0.025 per cent cream applied every other night. (If after four weeks there is no redness or flaking, it can be applied nightly; some people benefit from an increase to a 0.05 per cent strength. A dermatologist will advise.)

The face should be cleaned with a moisturising wash such as Cetaphil or Aquanil or pH 5.5 to reduce irritancy. Soaps or detergents should not be used as these dry the skin out more. A moisturiser (such as E45 cream, Eucerin, Vaseline or Nivea face creams) should be applied as required on the nights when Retin-A is not applied, and at other times in the day.

In addition, a broad-spectrum moisturising sunscreen (see page 112) should be applied every morning (in the UK and Europe, one that contains either Mexoryl SX or Tinosorb S, such as Ambre Solaire, Nivea Sun, Vichy, Roc, Soltan or Helios, and in the USA one that contains a stabilised form of Avobenzene, such as Oil of Olay, Shade UVA guard.

How should prescribed Retin-A be used?

For maximum benefits from Retin-A, treatment must be carried out regularly (nightly or every second or third night, depending on irritancy) for six months and then continued subsequently as part of a maintenance programme. This can be once weekly or 'weekend application'. Your dermatologist should provide you with a set of written instructions tailored specifically to your needs to help you to use it, but see the box above for my general advice to patients.

Myth Retin-A should not be used if you are going on holiday to a sunny destination because it increases sun damage.

Fact There is no evidence to suggest that Retin-A increases the risk of sun damage. I routinely prescribe it year-round in southern California and, in fact, if a sunscreen is used each morning and Retin-A is used nightly, there is a good chance that fewer sunspots will develop.

Another new retinoid cream/gel – Tazarotene

A new type of retinoid is Tazarotene cream or gel. It has been approved as a skin rejuvenation cream in the USA (called Avage Cream) and will hopefully soon be approved in Europe. Recent research shows that Tazarotene cream can reverse some of the effects of skin ageing much more quickly than Retin-A. My own experience using Tazarotene gel with my UK patients suggests that while the gel (approved for psoriasis) is also very effective, it can be more irritating than the cream (see below).

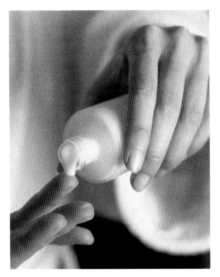

A rejuvenating prescription product, such as Retin-A or Tazarotene, has been proven to be effective.

How should Tazarotene cream or gel be used?

Tazarotene is used in a similar way to that described above for Retin-A, although, as it is more powerful, Tazarotene can be very slightly more irritating. The cream or gel is applied to the skin for ten minutes, then removed using a moisturising wash such as Cetaphil pH 5.5 or Dermol 500 in the UK or Cetaphil or Aquanil in the USA. The ten-minute contact time may be gradually increased over a period of several weeks, with some patients eventually leaving it on overnight. This gradual approach helps to reduce the risk of irritancy. As the gel tends to be more irritating than the cream, it is hoped that the cream will soon be available in Europe. Tazarotene has been used in the USA for acne and psoriasis for several years.

sunscreens

It is essential that you protect your skin as much as possible from the harmful effects of sunlight. The frequency of sunlight-induced skin ageing and skin cancers has been on the increase in most parts of the world. In particular, increasing numbers of melanoma skin cancer have been well documented in the last ten years. I feel that one possible explanation for this is that the older sunscreens we used to use (and in some instances still do!) did not offer adequate protection and that the documented increase in melanoma may therefore be due to past exposure to UVA as a result of inefficient sunscreens.

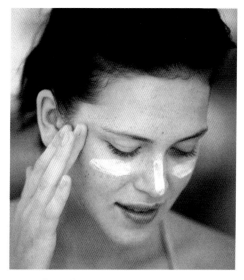

Use a broad-spectrum sunscreen in sufficient amounts.

Recent studies, including one carried out by British plastic surgeons, have suggested that using sunscreens may carry an increased risk of skin cancer. This is a dangerously misleading message to feed to the media; if there is an increased risk it is because people are being encouraged to stay out in the sun more because they are using sunscreen, rather than there being any inherent risk in the sunscreens themselves. My argument is that if the people stayed out of doors for

* * *   **Sunlight does have some health benefits...**   * * *

There is evidence that modest amounts of sun exposure can help to reduce the risk of certain diseases such as prostate cancer, psoriasis and multiple sclerosis, as well as in the prevention of osteomalacia (bone-thinning). Sun exposure should be kept to a minimum, however (no more than 20 minutes each day are necessary, and avoid exposure between the hours of 10am and 2pm during the summer months). Patients should have regular check-ups with a dermatologist if they have a risk of skin cancer. Assuming that these guidelines are followed, there should not be a problem with accelerated skin ageing or skin cancer, although people with either a personal or family history of skin cancers should not undergo therapeutic ultraviolet or sunlight treatment.

the same amount of time without the sunscreen, they would incur more severe sun damage and be more likely to develop skin cancer than if they had used protection.

A recent book published by an academic scientist in the USA suggested that there might be an advantage in exposing the skin to ultraviolet or sunlight because it is needed to form vitamin D, which is important for some diseases (see page 111). This suggestion went against all the accepted and well-tested theories of the risks of sun exposure causing skin cancers and skin ageing and led to the scientist being fired from his university. The chairman of his department stated 'that this was similar to suggesting that an excellent way of losing weight is to start smoking cigarettes'. You only require a very small amount of sun exposure to produce vitamin D (up to 20 minutes per day). All modern sunscreens, however, filter and do not completely block sunlight, therefore even the most protective sunscreens allow small amounts of ultraviolet through to give you adequate vitamin D synthesis.

Applying sunscreen

Sunscreen should be applied daily (after washing in the morning) to exposed parts of the skin. Apply at least a tablespoonful of sunscreen to the face and neck and half a tablespoon to your hands and allow it to dry for several minutes, giving it a chance to bind to the skin, before you get dressed (so that it does not rub off onto your shirt collar) or apply makeup. Do not apply a moisturiser since this will dilute the sunscreen, making it less effective; your sunscreen will act as a moisturiser instead.

What are the ingredients to look for in a sunscreen?

The most effective sunscreens are those that do not break down or degrade in sunlight. Two ingredients in European sunscreens that possess this stabilising effect are Mexoryl SX and Tinosorb S. They are usually incorporated with other ingredients (such as octocrylene, octylmethoxycinnamate and homosalate) to give a broad-spectrum sunscreen. The sun protection factor (SPF) tells you how much UVB protection. UVB + maximum UVA protection= broad-spectrum sunscreen.

What actually is an SPF?

An SPF – or sun protection factor – is a measure of how well a sunscreen protects the skin from sunburn; the higher the SPF, the better the protection. Maximum UVA protection is also important for all skin types as UVA is responsible for skin ageing, pigment spots and mask of pregnancy, as well as having some potential for increasing melanoma risk.

* * * Suggested SPF for Routine Outdoor Sun Exposure * * *

Skin Type*	Suggested SPF value
1	25–30 (waterproof)
2	25–30 (waterproof)
3	15 (waterproof)
4	15 (waterproof)
5	15 (waterproof)
6	15 (waterproof)

Always ensure that you:

- apply enough sunscreen – one tablespoon for the face and neck and half a tablespoon for the backs of hands – and let it dry for five minutes before dressing or applying makeup

- choose sunscreens with maximum UVA protection, regardless of skin type (in the UK, check the UVA star rating in which four stars denote maximum protection).

* See pages 28–29 to identify your own skin type.

In the USA, unfortunately neither Mexoryl SX nor Tinosorb S has as yet been approved, so choose sunscreens containing Avobenzene – also known as Parsol 1789. Some of these sunscreens, however, are not stable, but may be improved by combining Avobenzene with ingredients such as octocrylene, e.g. in Ombrelle, Oil of Olay and Shade UVA guard.

In principle, if a sunscreen is made by a reputable manufacturer (such as Boots, Eucerin, Garnier, Johnson & Johnson, L'Oréal, Olay, Piz Buin and Vaseline) it should have the right ingredients in the right concentrations. Those sunscreens containing the ingredients mentioned above offer very effective protection against UVB and, as importantly, UVA (see page 16). Evidence drawn from large population studies in Australia, for example, has confirmed that daily sunscreen use reduced the incidence of skin pre-cancers (solar keratoses). This is proof that daily use can reduce solar keratoses, which are the 'markers' of sun damage and, by extrapolation, are likely to reduce squamous cell cancers, which develop in 14 per cent of solar keratoses.

My personal preference when choosing a sunscreen is for a non-greasy spray-on variety that dries quickly and resists rub-off, as well as having high water-resistance properties, an SPF factor of 30 and UVA protection of three or four stars in the UK.

Valuable ingredients to look for in a sunscreen

UVA absorbers

Avobenzene – USA and worldwide

Mexoryl SX – worldwide, except for USA*

Tinosorb – worldwide, except for USA*

UVB-absorbing sunscreen chemicals

Methoxycinnamate – worldwide

Homosalate – worldwide

Octocrylene – worldwide

Sulfonic acid – worldwide

Tinosorb – worldwide, except USA*

Other important 'micronised powder' sunscreens

Titanium dioxide – worldwide

Zinc dioxide – worldwide

These absorb UVB and UVA and may be combined with the other ingredients listed above. These sunscreens have a whitish or powdery appearance on the skin but may be coloured to encourage children and sportsmen to use them.

*Correct as at September 2004.

Sunscreens in other products

Unfortunately it is difficult to judge the usefulness of other products – some makeup and moisturisers, for example – claiming to offer sun protection because they are not developed and tested to the same standards as proper sunscreening products.

Sunless tans

'Fake tans'

These have been greatly improved over the years and would be my number-one recommendation to anyone who wants a tanned appearance. The essential ingredient in a 'fake tan' is dihydroxyacetone (DHA) which has been used for several decades. It 'tans' the outer stratum corneum (see page 12), and lasts approximately five days, after which the stratum corneum is shed by the skin.

While the older products used to smell, rather unfortunately, of roast pork, cosmetic companies have refined their products and some now have very pleasant fragrances. Some also come with special preparations to treat the skin before the self-tanning product is applied. These are important in helping to remove any loose, flaking areas of the stratum corneum and allowing the product to bind well and last as long as possible. Some good products include Ambre Solaire self-tanning creams for face and body, Decleor self-tanning products and St Tropez Instant Tanning System.

Sun-protective clothing

This is a great innovation that I would recommend if you or your children are going to be outdoors for prolonged periods. Companies such as Solumbra (USA) use specially woven materials for sun-protective clothing and hats.

Another idea is to soak outdoor clothing in a formula of Tinosorb sunscreen, which can work well with some fabrics, but less well on others. More research is needed.

Spray-on tans

A spray-on 'airbrush' tan – Sudo Tropical Tan – which can be sprayed over the entire body if desired, can produce a very attractive, uniform tan for those who want a suntanned appearance without the sun.

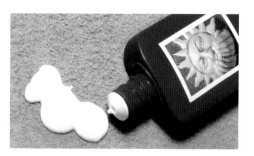

Sunscreens for children can also be coloured to aid even application.

Sun protection for children

There are safe sunscreen formulations for children, and they are usually labelled as such. These generally cause less irritation than the adult versions and may be used from the age of six months. Before this age it is best to use sun-protective clothing, including hats and prams or buggy hoods.

'Safe' tanning

There is no such thing as a safe suntan. Sunlight or UVA-induced tans are a sign that the skin has been damaged; they increase skin ageing, sunspots and skin cancer risks.

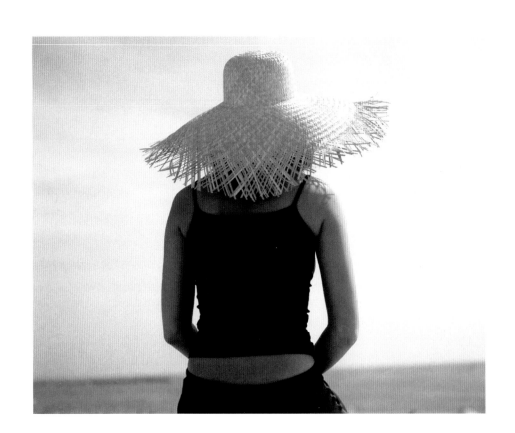

chapter five

lifestyle

Your lifestyle can impact considerably on how and at what stage your face and body begin to show signs of ageing. By looking at either one or both of your parents, you can sometimes form an idea of how you might look at a certain age. Often, there will be facial features in them that you recognise in yourself, and while some of these may be genetic, and therefore unavoidable, there will be others that you can control, perhaps by avoiding some of your parents' habits, such as smoking, drinking, overeating, crash dieting or sun-worshipping for example.

By making informed lifestyle choices, you can help to reduce the speed with which your face ages and develops problems such as spider veins and smoker's lines. How your face looks is governed significantly by the way you live. If you exercise regularly, eat healthily, drink plenty of water, stop smoking and reduce your alcohol intake, not only will you feel better, but this improvement will be reflected in your face.

Similarly, your daily cleansing routine and the creams and lotions you choose can also greatly affect your skin. Should you 'cleanse, tone and moisturise'? What if you have oily or dry skin? Does exfoliation help? And for men, what about shaving?

This chapter deals with ways in which you can improve your lifestyle with a view to delaying the onset of facial changes as you get older.

sun protection

For detailed information on sun protection, see chapter 4; however, suffice it to say here that natural or non-tanned skin is beautiful. A sunlight-induced tan leaves skin with cells that have been altered genetically and consequently prone to accelerated skin ageing and/or skin cancers. In particular, teenagers and younger adults find it difficult to believe that tanning themselves during their younger years can result in

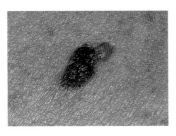

A malignant melanoma can be cured if treated early.

problems later, but this really is the case, although the effects may not become apparent until as long as 15 to 20 years after the sun exposure. It is important, therefore, to get the message through so that sun-worshipping teenagers do not find themselves with wrinkles, sagging skin, brown spots, spider veins, pre-skin cancers and cancers (including the potentially fatal melanoma) in their 20s and 30s and later in life. So, if it's a tan you are after, use one of the several excellent sunless tanning lotions or sprays (see box on opposite page).

Protecting your skin against the sun does not mean becoming a recluse. Use broad-spectrum sunscreens (see page 112) each morning and if you are on holiday swim either before 10am or after 3pm. Between those hours it is advisable to sit in a shady area, wearing sunscreen and a sun hat with a broad brim. The picture on the inside back flap of this book is a great illustration of

* * * **Melanoma** * * *

If you have a mole that shows any change, whether in size, colour or contour, or if it becomes itchy, crusted, scabbed or bleeds you must consult a dermatologist immediately. I would also recommend yearly skin check-ups if you have any family member with a history of melanoma, if you have multiple moles or if you suffered severe sunburn in your early years.

Note: a dermatologist is the optimally trained specialist to diagnose moles or melanoma correctly. Melanoma need not be fatal but **early** detection and removal are vital.

* * * Sun protection: the myths and the facts * * *

Myth You don't need to use sunscreens on cloudy or rainy days in summer or in winter or when driving in a car.

Fact Research has shown that even on a rainy day or when you are sitting in a car, long-wave ultraviolet (UVA, which is associated with skin ageing and increased risk for certain skin cancers) can penetrate through to your skin (see photograph below). The answer is to use a broad-spectrum sunscreen (see page 112) as a morning moisturiser, particularly if you have a risk of facial skin pigment (e.g. mask of pregnancy, see page 56) or a high risk of skin cancer.

how my granddaughter Annie and I were still able to enjoy a trip to Hawaii while taking all the necessary sun precautions.

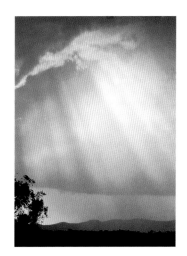

Sunlight-related ageing signs include:

- accelerated wrinkling and sagging

- spider veins and thread veins

- sallowness and brown sunspots

- precancerous solar keratoses, skin cancers including melanoma, some skin and internal diseases such as lupus erythematosus and sunlight-induced drug allergies

* * * Some good sun products * * *

Good sunscreen products
*with SPF 15 to 30 UVA, *** or ****

- Ambre Solaire
- Garnier
- L'Oréal
- Nivea Sun
- Roc

Good self-tanning
(sunless tanning products)

- DeCleor
- Fake Bake
- L'Oréal
- San Tropez mousse and cream
- Sudo Tan (air-brush tan)

smoking

There is ample evidence that smoking increases skin ageing as I mentioned in chapter 1. A smoker in their 40s may have as many wrinkles as a non-smoker in their 60s because the chemicals in cigarettes reduce the skin's elasticity. This is compounded by the amount of squinting a smoker does to keep the smoke out of their eyes as well as the puckering around the mouth every time they drag on a cigarette.

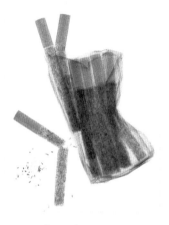

The only people who benefit are the tobacco companies.

The good news is, however, that there are numerous techniques and resources available to help you quit. (Incidentally, a recent study showed that cutting back on smoking is not enough; you really do have to quit completely.) Some of the modern nicotine-release patches and tablets can be extremely effective, as are treatments such as hypnotherapy which can be tailored for specific addictions and disorders (I myself gave up smoking this way). Southern California leads the way against smoking, with fewer than 18 per cent of the whole population still doing it!

Special smoking prevention programmes play a vital role in educating the young and in helping to deliver the message that not only does smoking seriously damage your health, causing lung, heart and blood disease, it also carries a very high risk of making you look much older than your years.

* * * **Smoking-related ageing signs** * * *

Smoking can cause the following changes in your skin:

- wrinkling
- sagging
- lines around the lips
- crow's feet
- sallowness

- cold, white, old-looking fingers, caused by blood-vessel damage
- a blue, bloated appearance and abnormal nails, caused by lung disease

stress

Repetitive stress can in itself lead to accelerated ageing as well as causing you to turn to habits such as comfort eating, smoking, drinking and other addictions which carry their own risks. A recent study reported that facial acne in female university students worsens around the time of examinations and this can be a factor in increasing facial ageing.

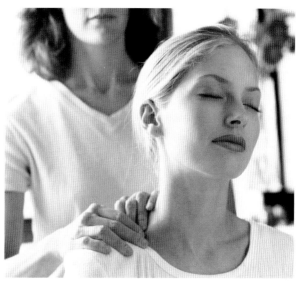

Relaxation not only helps improve your skin, it has many other health benefits. Take time out for yourself.

Sleep deprivation can also add to an increasingly tired and older look, for example eyelid sagging and bags under eyes. An on-going lack of sleep as a result of mood changes, anxiety or depression can become self-perpetuating, causing increased stress levels, worsening skin diseases such as eczema and psoriasis and producing less and less restful sleep. Stress management techniques, hypnotherapy, yoga and exercise are all helpful. You should be able to find classes and a reputable practitioner, where applicable, to help you with these techniques. There are also many good books available on stress management. In some cases physician-prescribed medication may be required. Never be afraid to seek professional help.

* **Stress-related ageing signs** *

Stress can cause the following changes in your skin:

- increased frown lines (worry lines)
- acne
- hair loss

alcohol

Consumed in modest quantities (two glasses of wine daily or equivalent) alcohol is unlikely to result in any skin or facial problems. However people who are susceptible to facial flushing may want to reduce or stop drinking alcohol in order to reduce the likelihood of their developing facial spider and thread veins. It is when larger amounts of alcohol are imbibed that the problems with health and appearance begin. Excess drinking leads to rapidly changing levels in fluid retention, which in turn alters the way in which blood vessels behave, causing spider veins and bloating. In the more advanced stages of alcohol abuse the liver becomes damaged and cannot expel toxins efficiently, causing more bloating and yellow-looking skin and eyes. And of course, your general health is at stake as well as your appearance.

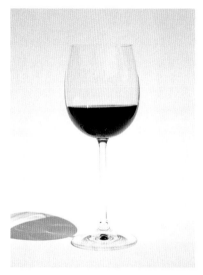

A little red wine may be good for your heart, but too much can cause spider and thread veins.

Help is at hand for anyone who feels they have a problem with alcohol, and recognising that there is a problem is the first important step. Ask your GP for suggestions or contact Alcoholics Anonymous (AA). This is an incredibly supportive and successful worldwide organisation through which countless people have conquered their addiction.

* * * **Alcohol-related ageing signs** * * *

Alcohol can cause the following changes in your skin:

- spider veins
- thread veins
- bloating
- sallowness

exercise

A young appearance is dependent not only on your face, but also on your body and, in particular, your fitness level and attitude to life. Regular exercise is very important in helping to prevent obesity. At the same time it is also a great outlet for stress, leads to good skin oxygenation (which improves skin colour and tone) and engenders an overall feeling of vitality. However, exercise alone cannot fight the ageing process; it must be adopted along with other appropriate lifestyle changes (see my other suggestions in this chapter) if it is to be beneficial for general health maintenance, a positive outlook and, by extension, the way you look.

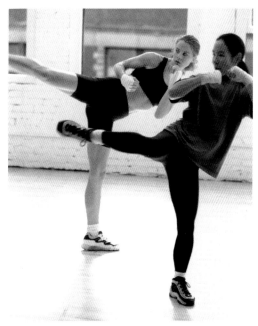

Many of us find it difficult to make time for regular exercise but making a commitment is half the battle. Why not start by taking a walk at lunchtime? Walking, tennis, swimming and exercise machines are all good options. One of my own best lifestyle choices was to see a personal trainer, who has helped to start me off and maintain a programme of regular exercise. I have lost weight, feel more dynamic and have even been told that I look younger!

Try to do about 30 minutes of light exercise, 5 times a week – even if it is hoovering or walking the dog.

* * * Lack-of-exercise-related ageing signs * * *

Lack of exercise can cause the following changes in your skin:

- poor circulation
- sallowness
- fat accumulation on chin and jowls
- bloated appearance

diet

An enormous amount has been written over the years about the best foods to eat in order to prevent ageing of the body. Many diets have turned out to be no more than fads and have not stood the test of time. Some mysteriously seem to re-emerge with a different title but very similar content, claiming to be new, 'breakthrough' diets. With all this information vying for the public's attention, it comes as no surprise, therefore, that we have become almost obsessed with what, when and how we eat, and that diet and cookery books seem to occupy a permanent place in the bestseller lists.

Can our diet affect our facial appearance?

Diet can affect our looks in several ways. As I have said earlier, acne can contribute to ageing of the skin by increasing the breakdown of elastic and collagen tissue and recent studies have shown that excess carbohydrates (such as white sugar, chocolate and sweets) can exacerbate this condition (see pages 34–35). It has been shown that by lowering your intake of refined sugars by about 10 per cent, you can decrease the action of those hormones responsible for making the skin oily and this in turn can reduce acne. Researchers involved in these studies also commented that in societies where very little processed food is eaten acne is extremely rare. I believe that, as this study suggests, diet is a factor in some acne-prone people, although further research into this link is needed.

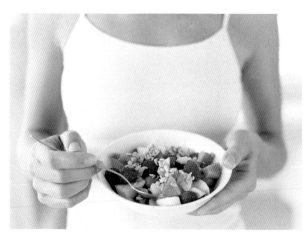

You are what you eat – and it is reflected in the way you look. A varied diet of healthy foods, each taken in moderation, will help your skin.

It is also certainly true to say that crash or obsessive dieting can make the face look more drawn and gaunt with increased lines and a generally older appearance because of the loss of some of the supportive fat under the skin. Even well-known popular diets such as the Atkins diet can have this effect because they

Dietary recommendations

- Cut back on your overall amount of food intake. Most people in the western world eat more food than they need to maintain good health – if you feel hungry, try small healthy snacks (fruit or nuts).

- Keeping a food diary can be helpful in estimating the number of calories you are eating each day.

- Reduce your intake of saturated fats, found typically in red meat, butter and ice cream. Also look out for trans fats, found in processed foods, margarines and many packaged meals, which may actually be more dangerous than saturated fats.

- Cut back on simple carbohydrates such as white bread and sugar.

- Eat plenty of beans, nuts, grains and cereals.

- Eat at least 5 portions of fruit and vegetables a day as they are good sources of vitamins and antioxidants, but beware, vitamin C is fragile and one study found that levels dropped dramatically in orange juice after 8 days in the fridge.

- Allow yourself times, around Christmas and Thanksgiving, for example, when you will eat more of what is not good for you, but plan the rest of your eating routine so that such periods of overindulgence can be happily accommodated.

- Drink plenty of non-caffeinated, non-alcoholic fluids – preferably water! – to ensure good urine output. This helps to maintain good toxin clearance and also to avoid dehydration. It is particularly important where there is low humidity (i.e. hot, dry weather) or central heating, during exercise and on long-haul flights.

will produce the classic early signs of rapid weight loss that I have already described. In the early fat-burning (ketotic) phase of the Atkins diet many people look grey, pallid and generally older and unhealthy.

Obesity, on the other hand, also takes its toll on facial appearance. It increases jowl size, creates a double chin effect and also causes extra fat pads under the eyes. These all combine to produce an older-looking individual.

These are just some of the ways in which our faces can be directly affected by what we do (or do not) eat. It is therefore important for all of us to follow sensible eating guidelines, not only for our overall health but also to benefit our facial appearance.

good dietary habits

One of the first things that comes to mind when looking at eating habits is quantity. In general, in the developed world food portions are far too generous from a health as well as facial ageing point of view. This is particularly noticeable in parts of the United States, where obesity has become a major problem. Interestingly it is less evident in southern California, possibly because there is such a strong emphasis there on looking youthful, fit and attractive.

Another important factor is how well balanced our diet is. Let's take a look now at the various food types, and how they can affect our skin.

Carbohydrates

These may be divided into simple 'fast-acting' carbohydrates and complex or 'slow-release' carbohydrates.

Simple carbohydrates (found in sweets, chocolate, jam and desserts) release energy quickly into the body, often leaving us with a post-sugar 'crash' or a feeling of tiredness.

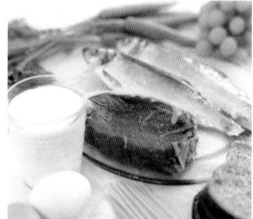

A balanced diet – complex carbs, lean meat, oily fish and fresh fruit and veg.

They will thus (indirectly) affect appearance and skin ageing through obesity. There has also been research to suggest that they may exacerbate acne (see pages 34–35).

Complex carbohydrates release their energy more slowly and are therefore more beneficial for general health. They are found in whole grains and fresh fruit and vegetables which also contain vitamins and antioxidants, important for healthy and youthful-looking skin. With all their numerous benefits, therefore, these foods should constitute around 50 per cent of your diet (although Atkins diet devotees will disagree as far as weight loss is concerned).

Protein

Proteins form an essential part of our diet. They provide us with the essential amino acids which are needed to build cells, including those in the skin. Because the skin, hair and nails are highly active (they produce and turn over cells very quickly) it is very important to ensure that they are 'fed' enough proteins to keep them healthy. Proteins also play a vital role in the formation of collagen and elastin which, as we have seen, are essential for youthful-looking skin.

Good sources of protein include lean meat, fish, eggs, cheese, beans, peas, soy and lentils, and such foods should constitute between 15 and 25 per cent of your diet, for general health, good muscle tone and for your skin's needs. The Atkins and similar diets recommend a higher protein intake but it is unclear exactly how safe this balance is in the long term. There have been short-term studies (over one year) into this diet and it is clear that it does help people to lose weight; however no long-term studies into its effects on general health have been carried out as yet.

Fats

These are an important source of energy and are also important for healthy skin. They allow the skin to produce its own fats, or lipids, which act as an effective barrier against water loss (and therefore dry, scaling skin), making the skin feel smooth and supple.

However care should be taken to eat the right type of fats. It is best to eat fewer saturated fats (in red meat, butter and ice cream) and trans fats (in margarine and processed foods). Around 15–25 per cent of your diet should be made up of 'good' fats including omega-3 fats from oily fish. (See also page 129.)

Essential fatty acids (EFAs)

Because these cannot be manufactured by the body, it is vital that they form a part of our daily diet. They are found in foods such as vegetable oils, nuts and cereals. The most common EFAs are linoleic, linolenic and arachidonic acid and they are necessary for the normal working and functioning of the skin – forming, as they do, a key part of the skin barrier, as well as helping to control the speed at which healthy cells are produced.

EFA deficiency is not common and is unlikely to occur other than in cases of bowel disease, where there is a decrease in the absorption of fats and other nutrients, or in people suffering from severe starvation. When I carried out research into EFAs and the skin some 30 years ago for a doctoral thesis, I thought that they could be useful in the correction of common dry skin problems. In actual fact, the application of EFAs to the skin in, for example, sunflower seed oil, is not helpful, other than in cases of EFA deficiency which is very rare.

Essential fatty acids, such as evening primrose oil supplement capsules, are important in maintaining an adequate lipid supply in the epidermis, although they are no longer thought to be of benefit in treating atopic eczema.

Beans, nuts, cereals and grains

These foods are known to be high in protein, vitamins (in particular B, which is necessary for the healthy formation of skin, hair and nails) minerals and fibre.

Dietary supplements

There are many supplements, including oral vitamins, minerals, marine extracts and antioxidants, that are said to have rejuvenative properties. However, there is not a lot of evidence to back this up. A study carried out in France suggested that oral supplements of vitamins A, C and E helped to prevent some skin ageing changes and damage from sunlight, although these findings have not been confirmed by other researchers.

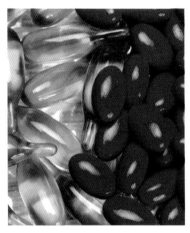

Dietary supplements can back up your diet.

My recommendation is to take a multi-vitamin, mineral and antioxidant supplement once a day, which will provide you with the recommended daily amounts of these nutrients. Several of these are available in pharmacies – ask your pharmacist if in doubt. Reliable brands include Boots, One-A-Day, Sanatogen, Solgar and Centrum.

* * * **Biotin** * * *

Biotin is usually classed as one of the vitamin B group and can be taken orally. It has beneficial effects on the nails – studies using biotin have been shown to improve nail brittleness and peeling – and may also be important for the formation of hair. It has been used for many years as a supplement to prevent horses' hooves from cracking and thus from our veterinary colleagues we have learned that biotin can improve keratin-derived structures like hooves, nails and hair! A daily supplement containing biotin could help to improve the quality of your hair and nails.

fighting ageing with fish?

There has been a lot of talk recently about the possibility that we might fight the ageing process by consuming large amounts of oily fish. Oily fish (and some shellfish) contain high levels of the omega-3 fatty acids, often described as 'good' fats. (Incidentally, some brands of hens' eggs now contain high levels of these fatty acids and are being promoted as healthy, 'smart' eggs.) Omega-3 fatty acids have been shown to reduce inflammation in blood vessels and in conditions such as arthritis. So, the theory goes that by reducing inflammation because they are high in antioxidants (which help to 'mop up' free radicals), they may also help to reduce the rate at which our skin ages. However, there is, as yet, insufficient scientific evidence to back up this theory and while I myself love to eat sardines, herrings, salmon and all types of seafood, I do not think they make me look younger! However, having said that, I have heard that those who follow the recommendations of a recent skin book advocating a diet that is rich in oily fish may not need to worry about how they look as few people will want to go near them because of their fishy odour!

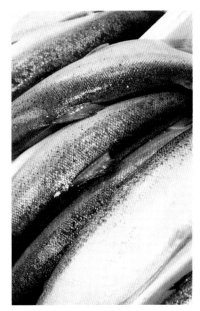

Oily fish is good for your body, but may not reduce skin ageing.

There are also recent fears that certain fish can concentrate poisons (toxins) in their muscles and in particular there is concern regarding the levels of mercury that have been found in a variety of fish, including tuna and swordfish. Also, farmed salmon seems to be more risky from certain sources than wild salmon – it all depends on what and where the fish are farmed. It is thought that small fish such as sardines are likely to be safer because they contain low levels of toxins. Sensible recommendations are as follows:

- children and pregnant or nursing women should avoid swordfish, shark, tuna and marlin altogether

- eat fish in moderation – no more than 140g per week for children and pregnant/nursing women and 340g per week for healthy adults (World Health Organisation recommendations, *Time* magazine, 8 December 2003)

- buy your fish from a reputable store or supplier who can vouch for its origins.

skin-care routines

With so many companies competing to sell a huge range of different skin products, it is hardly surprising that many of us feel confused and unsure as to the best skin-care routine to adopt. Although expensive and impressive advertising, along with media hype, often lead us to believe that a given product is the last word in skin care, there is often a worrying absence of scientific information available to back up their claims.

The answer, I think, is to keep things as simple and as practical as possible, but before deciding on a daily skin-care routine, you need to address the following key questions:

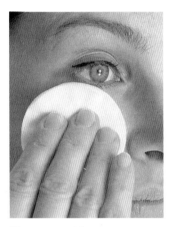

Keep your skin-care routine simple.

- how does your skin respond to different stimuli and cleansers? In other words, would you say you have sensitive skin, oily skin, dry skin, normal skin or a combination skin (see box, right, to help you identify your own skin type)?

- do you have eczema, psoriasis, acne or any condition that is likely to increase your skin's response to products?

Your dermatologist will be able to help you to identify your skin type. Once you have established which type you are, you may follow the suggested skin-care routines on pages 135–137 but first, let's take a look at what these actually do.

Cleansing the eyes

This area needs careful treatment as eyelid skin is extremely thin and more sensitive to allergy and irritation. It also contains very few sebaceous (oil) glands and can therefore be prone to dryness. Eye cleansing products containing humectants such as glycerine and hyaluronic acid can help to prevent drying of the eyelid skin.

Cleansing

There are endless varieties of different cleansing lotions, soap bars, gels and washes. The secret is to identify your skin type, then simply to find one or two products that suit your skin and to stick with them.

If you have dry skin, you may find that you have to adjust your cleansing routine slightly according to the season and also to where you are as your skin can change in different environments. It is also important to avoid

* * * Skin types * * *

Sensitive skin Your skin will react to a variety of creams (some sunscreens, renewal creams, glycolic acid creams) by stinging or burning. You may have a personal or family history of eczema or other skin irritations. You need to use skin products that are tested and labelled specifically for sensitive skin.

Dry skin Your skin will often feel tight and 'stretched'. You usually do not have any oily areas on your face and you may have some patches of flaking skin. You need to use non-soap, moisturising washes. Your skin may often also be sensitive and you may not be able to tolerate renewal creams, at least not frequently.

Normal skin Your skin feels neither greasy nor dry, which means you are fortunate to have a whole range of skin-care products available to you.

Oily skin Your skin feels greasy or oily and often looks shiny, particularly on the forehead. You may be prone to oil bumps (sebaceous hyperplasia – yellow or white bumps under the skin) as you age. You need to use degreasing cleansers and toners and sometimes oil-absorbing face masks. The good news is that your skin is unlikely to be sensitive and can tolerate many creams, including renewal creams.

Combination skin Your skin is a combination of oily (usually on the forehead and nose – the T-zone, where there are more sebaceous glands) and normal or dry (more often the cheeks and around the mouth and neck). Different cleansing routines are needed for the different areas, or products aimed specifically at combination skin types. Up to 50 per cent of women have combination skin.

overcleansing as this can cause your skin to dry out even more. Your objective when cleansing is simply to remove surface dirt, makeup and the day's creams. Use a gentle sweeping motion, rather than powerful rotary movements.

For more oily skin, cleansing (and toning) can be very helpful, particularly for removing some of the blackheads and whiteheads that can be characteristic of this skin type. However, you should try to cleanse only the oily areas. Cleansing masks, some of which contain kaolin or bentonite clay, can also be beneficial, but again should only be used on oily areas. They can be too drying in other skin areas.

Toning

Toning is more important if you have a tendency to dull or oily skin because it helps to clean the skin and reduces surface oils. But if your skin is dry, you should avoid toning, or reduce the frequency. Some botanical ingredients, for example aloe vera and avocado oils, are good moisturisers; others such as tea-tree oil may be good against skin infections because of their antiseptic qualities.

Moisturising

For sun-exposed skin, for example the face, neck and hands, use your sunscreen as a moisturiser (see pages 112–113, 118–119). If you have dry, flaking skin, moisturising will help to reduce dryness by preventing further water loss from your skin and your skin will look smoother and feel softer. It is also better than scrubbing. Be careful not to overmoisturise if you have oily or acne-prone skin.

Night creams

It is always important to moisturise the face and around the eyes before you go to sleep because moisturisers tend to work more efficiently at night than during the day because the stratum corneum barrier is less exposed at night, allowing your moisturiser to stay in contact more readily than during your daily activities.

* * * Cleansers vs soap and water * * *

There is an on-going debate as to whether we are better off using designated cleansers or simply soap and water. The measure we use to gauge acidity or alkalinity is known as pH – a pH of less than 7.5 is acidic, whereas above that figure it is more alkaline. The skin's pH is around 5.5, i.e. it is naturally slightly acidic – you may have heard the term 'acid mantle' used to describe the protective acidic barrier (pH5.5) with which the skin protects your body. Most detergent soaps are more on the alkaline side and tend to be harmful to the skin because they destroy the skin's natural balance. They can also cause irritation. Many of the modern, soap-free, pH-balanced cleansers, on the other hand, have a pH of around 5.5 (the same as that of normal skin), which makes them perfect for cleansing and protecting.

Skin exfoliation is always a contentious subject. While gentle exfoliation can help the skin to look more alive and healthy, do not forget that besides removing damaged skin cells, it can also remove some of the protective cells from the skin surface. Avoid harsh exfoliants such as Brasivol (unless you have acne and do not have sensitive skin); sometimes alpha-hydroxy acid lotions, which can loosen the cement between the surface cells are enough to exfoliate without producing excess dryness.

Exfoliate occasionally if your skin is rough, and probably not at all if you have dry skin.

To conclude, remember the golden rule of skin care: keep your routine as simple and regular as possible. Do not keep adding or experimenting with new and different products as you might end up exposing your skin to problems such as dryness, irritancy, allergy or acne quite unnecessarily. Once you have found the combination that works for you, stay with it – as they say, 'if it ain't broke, don't fix it.'

shaving

Shaving is necessary for most men and some women. It can be a traumatic process for the skin and a moisturising shaving cream can help to lessen skin damage. A post-shaving moisturiser is also advisable. Try to shave when your skin is softer, often after bathing.

Electric shavers can be more gentle than blade razors because they are designed to cut the hair shaft close to the skin surface but not actually scrape the skin, which can cause skin damage. It may take several days of electric shaving for your skin to feel smooth.

If you are prone to shaving rash, avoid soap and use a moisturiser. If that doesn't work, apply a half per cent strength (over-the-counter) hydrocortisone cream, and if it still doesn't improve, consult a dermatologist.

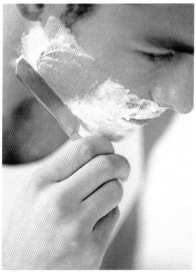

Moisturising before shaving will help soften the hair.

✳ ✳ ✳ Examples of well-tested products ✳ ✳ ✳

The following products may help to reduce some fine lines, but in the long term, their skin rejuvenation effects will not be as good as those of prescription creams. All the products mentioned here have been well tested for safety because of the well-guarded reputation of their companies.

Some non-prescription creams with skin rejuvenation potential

Avene, L'Oréal Visible Results Ultra Smoothing Day Cream, L'Oréal Wrinkle Decreasing Cream, L'Oréal Wrinkle De-Crease Serum, Luminous Eye Care, Marks and Spencer Revival Complex, Neutrogena Copper Visibly Young Eye and Face Cream, Nivea Visage, Nivea Moisture Body Boost, Nivea Age Reversal Night Cream, Olay Total Effects Cream, Olay Regenerist Serum, Roc Retin-Ox Lotion, Roc Retin-Ox Correction, Vaseline Dermacare.

Some 'gentle' face and eye moisturising creams for sensitive skin

Aqueous cream BPC, Aveeno cream, Boots E45 cream, Diprobase, Neutrogena facial moisturiser, Nivea Age Renewal Night Cream, Nivea Visage and eye creams, Olay facial moisturiser, Olay Luminescence, Vaseline Intensive Care, L'Oréal face and eye moisturisers. Dermol 500 Lotion can be used as a moisturiser and a wash – very useful for eczema and dry skin.

Don't waste your money on expensive products – spend it on a good dermatology consultation!

✳ ✳ ✳ DIY skin care ✳ ✳ ✳

- *Cucumbers on the eyelids* If you have puffy eyelids from too much partying (or before a period) cucumber slices on the eyelids can help to reduce fluid build-up by withdrawing some of the fluid from the skin through osmosis. They also feel refreshing, particularly straight from the refrigerator.

- *Teabags on the eyelids* These have a similar effect to that of cucumbers but make sure they have cooled down sufficiently before applying. Alternatively keep some ready-soaked teabags in the refrigerator.

- *Avocados* Not only delicious, they can also make a good moisturising cream as they contain excellent moisturising oils.

facial skin-care routines

For dry and sensitive skin

Morning

1. Cleanse, using water plus pH-neutral non-soap cleanser, e.g. ph5.5 Cetaphil or Dermol 500.

2. Dry gently.

3. Do not use toner.

4. Apply sunscreen (ideally a moisturising variety) and allow to dry for 10 minutes.

5. Apply makeup if desired.

Evening

1. Cleanse using water plus a non-soap cleanser as above.

2. Use a rejuvenation cream (see top box on opposite page). You may only be able to tolerate this once or twice a week and you may need to avoid it altogether at certain times of the year, for example in dry winters, in which case use a gentle moisturiser instead. If you want to use a prescription-strength rejuvenation cream, ask your dermatologist for Retin-A at 0.025 per cent (lower strength) or Tazarotene 0.05 per cent and rinse off after 10 minutes to reduce irritancy. Your skin may only be able to tolerate these every third or fourth night, so use gentle moisturising night creams for the face and eyes on alternate nights.

For normal moisturised skin

Morning

1. Wash with non-soap cleanser or moisturising milk or lotion.

2. Dry.

3. Apply sunscreen and allow to dry for ten minutes.

4. Apply makeup if desired.

No moisturiser needed – use your sunscreen as a moisturiser.

Evening

1. Wash as in the morning.

2. Dry.

3. Apply prescription Retin-A or Tazarotene cream for ten minutes (see page 110). If redness occurs, use less frequently (every second or third night). Your skin should become tolerant to these within seven to ten days. Weaker, non-prescription 'retinoid' creams are available, such as Avéne or Roc Retinol products.

4. Use moisturising face and eye cream as needed.

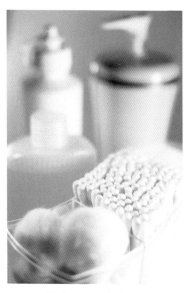

Make sure that you choose products to suit your skin type.

For combination skin

This is a very common skin type (see page 131), often accompanied by blackheads and whiteheads on the nose and central cheeks.

Morning

1. Wash with soap-free cleanser for combination skin.

2. Pat dry.

3. Use a moisturiser on sides of face and neck if they are dry.

4. Allow to dry.

5. Apply a light, non-greasy sunscreen (e.g. a sunscreen spray or light lotion).

6. Apply makeup if desired.

Evening

1. Use same cleanser as in the morning.

2. Allow to dry for at least ten minutes.

3. You may use prescription Retin-A or Tazarotene cream (or a weaker, non-prescription alternative such as Avene or Roc Retinol products) for the central oily area, but avoid any dry skin areas.

4. Apply moisturising cream to dry areas.

5. Apply moisturising eye cream.

For oily skin

This skin type can become more oily in hot, humid weather and less so in winter and climates with low humidity. (Sometimes oily skin may become combination skin in the winter, in which case, see left.) Oily skin is generally more tolerant of treatments such as Retin-A cream.

Morning

1. Wash with cleanser for oily skin. You may want to use an oil-absorbing mask occasionally.

2. Pat dry.

3. Apply an oil-free, light sunscreen.

You may wish to repeat this routine around lunchtime if your skin is very oily.

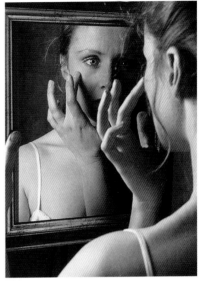

Use a mirror to apply creams accurately – this applies to men as well as women.

Evening

1. Wash with cleanser for oily skin.

2. Dry.

3. Use an oil-absorbing mask on some evenings if your skin is very oily as long as it does not cause irritation.

4. Apply an alcohol-based toner.

5. Dry.

6. Apply prescription Retin-A or Tazarotene cream or a good night cream.

You may also wish to wash and use a mask and toner before going out to an evening function or party. Some makeup, e.g. powder-based products such as Jane Iredale, will act as an oil absorber.

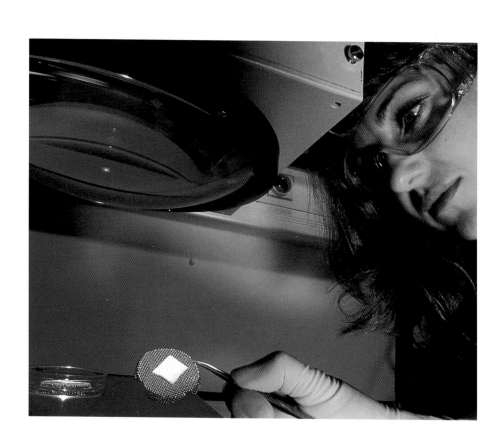

chapter six

the future

Already we have seen things happen that were almost unimaginable not that long ago: Restylane and Perlane (see pages 79–82) have made huge inroads in the treatment of nasolabial folds, lines on the face and sunken scars; in the last two to three years, skin renewal fillers such as NewFill (see page 83) have enabled us to stimulate new growth of the dermis, producing long-term improvements in lines and scars; and non-ablative treatment with lasers (see pages 62–63) and light are now used very successfully to rejuvenate the skin without the inconvenience of peeling, burning and the time taken for healing.

But what of the future? The following is a pot-pourri of my own thoughts and predictions as to how skin rejuvenation treatments and techniques will continue to improve and develop for the benefit of the population. With my crystal ball, I can envisage several areas in which breakthrough treatments are set to emerge:

- **New technology in cosmetics.** Companies are constantly coming up with new names and descriptions of their products so that they can tempt us to believe they have a special magic ingredient that will correct the fading and ageing of our skin. Some of these are genuine advances, for example the field of so-called nanotechnology, where very small particles surround an ingredient to encourage it to penetrate more deeply into your skin. There are some benefits with antioxidants and rejuvenating ingredients, such as vitamin E, tocopherol, vitamin C, vitamin A derivatives, e.g. retinol palmitate. Some of the newer ingredients include chemicals such as growth factors. These are frequently large molecules that have difficulty penetrating the skin. The idea is that they will promote the growth of new collagen and elastic tissue thereby making the skin more youthful. We want these to get into the dermis and nanotechnology will help them to do so. Microspheres have a similar effect and have been around for several years.

One of the potential problems of these very nano-sized particles is that they can penetrate the skin more than you actually want. One concern is that it is not known whether some of the sunscreen ingredients, e.g. titanium dioxide and zinc oxide, are safe if allowed to penetrate the skin too deeply and it has been shown that some very small particles containing sunscreens can end up inside your body, even in the lymph glands. They may therefore enter other organs and could cause diseases such as cancer, so the safety issues need to be thoroughly investigated. In fact, this whole area of improved delivery of cosmetic ingredients needs to be closely examined by the safety toxicology experts.

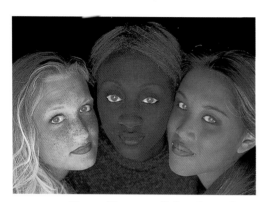

Three skin types, lit by ultraviolet light, showing different melanin amounts in the skin. From left to right: caucasian, black and Asian.

• **Better combination creams** that will be less irritating and more effective for skin rejuvenation. I expect that these will incorporate a combination of existing ingredients such as retinoids (as in Retin-A and Tazarotene) and some of the newer repair systems. These include the anti-oxidant superoxide dismutase (SOD) and Idebenone. Creams are currently being developed to repair damage done to the DNA in the skin by sunlight. They could be combined with regular morning sunscreens to prevent damage during the day.

• **Improved sunscreens.** These will afford greater protection because they will bind to and stay on the skin better. They will also contain ingredients to help in the repair of damage caused by small amounts of sunlight that have previously penetrated. I predict that these new highly protective sunscreens will, in the future, be combined with some of the repair systems that I have mentioned above as protective and rejuvenating creams.

• **Stimulating the skin to protect itself against the sun** may become a possibility by 'tricking' the genes into producing more protective melanin. This could help to reduce sun-induced skin ageing and skin cancers.

There is on-going research into improving the skin's own protection by increasing the melanin, which is the skin's protective tanning chemical. Melanin is a natural substance produced by the pigment cells (melanocytes) in the outer living skin or epidermis. There are two types of melanin: eumelanin, which occurs in most light- and dark-brown- and black-haired individuals; and phaeomelanin, which occurs in red-haired people. Eumelanin is very efficient at producing a tanned skin. This tan can protect from some, but not all, sunlight damage by absorbing the ultraviolet part of sunlight. In addition melanin acts to 'scavenge' or mop up the damaging products, e.g. free radicals that are produced in the skin in response to sun exposure. Redheads, on the other hand, do not have this type of protective eumelanin and are therefore more prone to sun damage. Recent research has shown that the genes that control the amount of melanin can be activated, but this approach requires further safety testing.

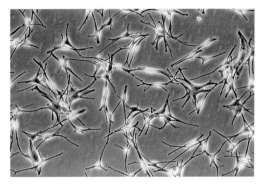

Research in cell culture systems will lead to improved skin renewal.

Studies are being planned on a hormone that stimulates tanning, reduces appetite and increases libido. If it proves safe and effective, it is likely to be rather popular!

- **Advances in techniques for computer-analysing skin types** will help to identify and recommend appropriate treatments. A computer-based assessment of the skin surface may enable us to predict the skin's response to a given product, for example Retin-A. It may even be able to gauge the level of sun damage the skin has sustained in the past and, based on this, predict the changes that are likely to occur. Again, this allows the dermatologist to formulate a tailored treatment plan.

- **New developments in skin injections** will result in improved capability to produce new collagen and elastin. NewFill has already paved the way forward and newer systems will combine cell cultures with growth factors to perform this job even more efficiently. This will lead to a whole new array of effective injectable skin fillers. There will be new injectable skin implants that will last for several years. These will be safer and more easily adjusted than permanent ones.

- **Progress in skin cell culture systems** will allow us to take tiny skin samples and then use them for rejuvenation of damaged skin. For example, we may treat damaged skin by laser and then seed the lasered areas with the cultured skin cells that will promote more youthful skin growth. This could also benefit people who have lost pigment as cell cultures may be taken from pigmented areas and similarly seeded where necessary. This would be a breakthrough for conditions such as vitiligo and for cases where scars have lost their pigment.

- **Hair cell culture techniques** are being developed and will eventually, I believe, allow us to take a small number of hair cells (possibly by hair plucking) which will then be grown and 'tricked' into producing hair that can then be transplanted back into the balding scalp.

- **Continued developments in the field of laser treatments** will achieve better, more uniform results. Blood vessel, pigment and hair removal lasers are already extremely accurate and efficient, and I predict that these and similar techniques will be extended to treat stretch marks.

- **Radiofrequency skin rejuvenation** is currently in the early stages of development (one system, Thermage, is already in clinical use in the USA). The idea is that it will target deeper areas of the skin, tightening skin beneath the skin surface to achieve rejuvenation of, for example, the forehead or the cheek area. This is an exciting development since, once perfected, this technology may offer a completely non-invasive approach to tightening sagging skin in several parts of the body.

- **Further research into radiofrequency and long wavelength laser devices** will, I believe, extend to reducing the activity of oil glands in the skin, thereby improving acne by reducing the amount of oil produced. This could be a breakthrough for those people whose acne is resistant to currently available treatments.

- **Continued work with Botox** could mean that it might, eventually, be used in creams and similar products. In its current form Botox will not work in a cream because the Botox molecule is too big to penetrate into the skin. With modern pharmacology techniques, however, it is conceivable that the active part of the Botox molecule could be made smaller and then, perhaps, be delivered more readily via patches, gels or micro current to the skin over the muscle areas that we wish to control. This, I must stress, is purely speculative at present.

- **Research into techniques for hair removal and greying hair** will receive considerable research effort. Improved treatments are needed for white and grey hair removal, particularly on the face. At the time of writing, none of the conventional hair removal lasers is successful in this respect as the laser is not absorbed by hair that does not contain any pigment, but it looks likely that a combination of new laser or light systems may be developed for the removal of white, grey or downy hair. These may be used with lotions or gels that absorb light. New oral medications to reduce the effects of hormones on the hair are also currently being developed. By identifying how to control the gene for greying hair, we could succeed in stopping the greying process. However, we are still a long way from turning theory into practice here.

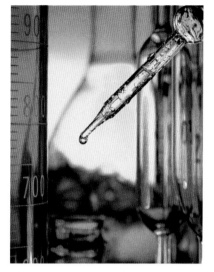

Collaboration between dermatology researchers, cosmetic, pharmaceutical and laser companies will lead to future breakthroughs.

- **Newer creams may be developed for hair removal** and also to reduce hair growth of all colours. I foresee further advances in this area because of the vast earning potential of this market to the cosmetic and pharmaceutical industry.

- **New developments in photodynamic therapy (PDT)** – a visible light-activated cream currently used to treat skin and pre-skin cancers – could make this a potential hair removal technique. Time and research will tell. Meanwhile, PDT has already advanced to the point that it can uniformly treat large areas of skin – for example, the whole face – in a single session. My prediction is that new, improved light-activated creams may be able to treat people with large areas of sun damage and thereby improve not only premature skin ageing, but also precancerous skin lesions beneath the skin surface. A whole new treatment area, in which I have been very involved, is being developed and is called skin photorejuvenating PDT treatment.

in conclusion

Demand for changes and improvements in rejuvenation treatments and techniques is on the increase, not least because more and more people in developed countries are living for longer and want to remain as youthful as possible. Advances in technology and research mean that techniques are constantly under review, evolving and progressing so that the dreams of just a few years ago are, as we have seen, already becoming a reality. With all this in mind, the future for skin rejuvenation looks very encouraging indeed.

appendix

choosing your practitioner

Dermatologists start out with full training at medical school for anywhere between five and eight years, depending on the country in which they are studying. Only then, having obtained a medical degree, can they begin training to become a specialist in the skin.

In the USA there are many recognised dermatology training programmes providing a broad spectrum of training and experience through which qualified medical dermatologists can then extend their knowledge and skills. The UCLA dermatology training programme, for example, where I have taught for the past 27 years, covers skills including serious disease dermatology (acne, psoriasis, blistering diseases and leprosy), skin cancers and melanoma as well as cosmetic surgery, laser treatment, liposuction and all current innovative rejuvenation treatments. There are currently in the USA around 9,000 dermatologists, about one third to one half of whom are fully trained and actively engaged in dermatologic surgery and cosmetic procedures. The American Society of Dermatologic Surgery has suggested that we call ourselves dermasurgeons to demonstrate this aspect of our speciality and to reduce the confusion in the general public about our skills (see page 146). A similar pattern may be seen in France, Italy, Spain and Germany, where a large proportion of qualified dermatologists have additional training in cosmetic procedures.

In the UK, however, the training of dermatologists has been largely determined by the budgetary rationing of the National Health Service. (Since 1948, in an effort to cut costs, the NHS has been rationing referrals to specialists – an initiative that has not, in fact, saved money but has led to inferior care.) Consequently, there are only about 450 dermatologists in the UK (around one for every 120,000 people, against one for every 30,000 in the USA), and, although a slow but growing number are beginning to branch out into dermatologic and cosmetic surgery, the focus of the majority is still confined to medical dermatology.

Finding a Practitioner

So, how to make sense of the web of names, titles, experts, non-experts, registers and associations in order to find the right person for the job? The task is somewhat easier, though not foolproof, in countries such as the USA, France, Italy, Spain and Germany than it is in the UK since, as we have seen, more qualified medical dermatologists in those countries have undertaken additional training in cosmetic procedures.

In the UK

In the United Kingdom you need to be particularly wary of specialist claims. The severe shortage in the UK of dermatologists and plastic surgeons has led a number of other people, for a variety of financial and other reasons, to practise cosmetic surgery, thereby creating a hazardous minefield of non-specialist, often even non-physician practitioners.

Ensure, therefore, that your chosen practitioner is a specialist-registered dermatologist or plastic surgeon with the General Medical Council as well as a member of the British Society for Dermatological Surgery. In addition, the British Association of Dermatology can provide you with information and has a list of trained dermatologists. The British Association of Aesthetic Plastic Surgeons can provide similar information about their specialists.

A trained British dermatologist will have the letters MRCP or FRCP after their name, denoting that they are a Member or Fellow of the Royal College of Physicians. A plastic surgeon, oculoplastic or head and neck surgeon will bear the initials FRCS (Fellow of the Royal College of Surgeons). Most also hold (or have previously held) a consultant appointment in the National Health Service.

In mainland Europe

In some European countries there are special training programmes for aesthetic medicine, which (for example in Italy) have proven to be a very satisfactory way of ensuring that the physician in question has undertaken special training. Physicians undergo several years of training in aesthetic or cosmetic procedures and should have certificates to prove their additional training. Some are now practising in the UK – ask for proof of their aesthetic training.

In the USA

A dermatologist in the USA who is board-certified in dermatology and a member of the American Society for Dermatologic Surgery should be able to provide you with evidence of special training in the procedures such as Botox, skin fillers, liposuction or hair transplantation. You should ask to see verification that they have attended relevant training seminars, as well as photographs showing patients they have treated. Also ask for the names of patients who would be willing to discuss their treatment with you. Some dermatologists are now called dermasurgeons, a term introduced by the American Society for Dermatologic Surgery in 2004. This term perfectly describes doctors with specialist training in dermatology in surgery. In the USA and many continental European countries such as France, Spain and Italy, there is a growing number of dermatologists who are also specialists in skin surgery, which includes skin cancers and cosmetic procedures.

Plastic surgeons should have attended an approved residency training programme, usually for at least four years. Again, this does not necessarily mean that they are skilled in all forms of treatment – further specialist training in cosmetic procedures is required.

For cosmetic eyelid surgery I strongly recommend using an ophthalmologic surgeon (an eye surgical specialist) who is registered with the American Board of Ophthalmology but who has also had additional training in ophthalmic plastic (oculoplastic) surgery.

Head and neck (also known as ear, nose and throat) specialists are excellent and many have been specially trained in plastic surgical procedures of the face. Make sure they are registered with the American Board of Otolaryngology (head and neck surgery) and have undertaken additional cosmetic procedure training.

What about the other people who offer cosmetic advice/treatment?

It is best to rely on the recommendations of a specialist to guide you. The financial benefits of work in this area are enticing and some clinics may not be staffed by specialist trained physicians and surgeons. (Interestingly, it is illegal in California and some other states for non-physician businessmen to run medical clinics.) Be sure to take expert advice and ask all the appropriate questions.

Non-medical qualified cosmetic 'experts'

Some of these non-medical specialists refer to themselves as cosmetic specialists or cosmetic skin specialists. These people may have previously worked with plastic surgeons and have, as a result of observing the surgeon, decided that they are equipped to offer consultations. It should be relatively easy to search these people out by asking direct questions about where they trained and in what speciality.

Bear in mind that some injections, such as Botox, are actually prescription drugs. These should only ever be given by a physician, or under a physician's direct supervision, which is clearly not the case where a nurse is working alone either at a Botox 'party', a home visit or a beauty salon.

Many beauty clinics offering laser or light therapy employ staff who do not have appropriate training, so be wary of these. This treatment should only be practised either by or under the guidance of a trained laser dermatologist or plastic surgeon.

Remember, cosmetic procedures are not a medical emergency and should be planned slowly and carefully. The importance of asking the right questions and taking your time before making any decision cannot be overstated.

What happens if things go wrong?

As I have stressed above and throughout the book, you are most likely to achieve a positive outcome to your treatment by choosing a trained specialist. However, this does not automatically mean that everything then goes according to plan.

The body is not a precise machine and can, in some cases, respond unfavourably to cosmetic procedures even when these are performed by specialist physicians and surgeons. Of course, if this does happen, if you have first ensured that you are in skilled hands, you will maximise your chances of successful correction.

Should a problem occur, my advice is always to return to your treating physician or surgeon. Often, when things go wrong, patients are tempted to seek advice elsewhere, but in fact it is the treating physician who is best informed about exactly what they have done and, assuming they are a trained specialist, they will be in a very good position to correct any problem that has arisen or to refer you to another specialist.

Titles and terms to be aware of when choosing a practitioner

Dermatologists

They need to be on the Specialist List of the General Medical Council (UK) or certified by the American Boards of Dermatology (USA). A dermatologist will have attended medical school for five to six years and then spent at least five to six years (UK) or three years (USA) at an approved dermatology training programme. In the UK they must have also first trained as internal general medical specialist and will be a Member (MRCP) or Fellow (more senior) of the Royal College of Physicians (FRCP). In the USA they will be a Fellow of the American Academy of Dermatology.

Dermatological surgeon, dermatological cosmetic surgeon, dermasurgeon

This is someone who has trained as a dermatologist (see above) and then has undertaken further training to include Botox, skin fillers, chemical peels, hair transplantation, laser surgery, liposuction, skin surgery and skin cancer treatment. This training will be as a Fellowship or part of a series of training sessions with experts.

Plastic surgeon

A physician who has then trained in surgery and spent five to six years (UK) or three to four years (USA) at an approved plastic surgery programme where they will have trained in reconstructive surgery. They may have additional speciality training in the aesthetic (cosmetic) branch of plastic surgery. In the UK they will be on the Specialist List of the General Medical Council and a Fellow of the Royal College of Surgeons (FRCS). In the USA they will be certified by the American Board of Plastic Surgery.

Aesthetic plastic surgeons

As for plastic surgeons (see above), but they will then have acquired extra experience in cosmetic surgery. They may have taken Fellowship training in aesthetic plastic surgery, e.g. liposuction, facelift, breast augmentation.

Head and neck cosmetic surgeon

A physician who has then trained as a surgeon with expertise in different types of head and neck surgery, more common in the USA than the UK. Must be on the Specialist List registered with the General Medical Council (UK) or certified by American Boards of Head and Neck Surgery (USA). In the UK they will have FRCS with specialist training.

Oculoplastic (opthalmic plastic) surgeon

A physician who has subsequently trained in surgery, they will have trained in ophthalmic surgery (five to six years in the UK or three to four years in the USA) then undergone additional training in plastic surgery of the eyelids, eyebrows and forehead. In the UK they will have FRCS with special expertise in ophthalmic surgery and be on the Specialist Register of the General Medical Council. In the USA they will be registered with the American Board of Ophthalmology.

All the above consultants and specialists are fully trained and should be the most competent to treat your cosmetic needs. In the UK they should hold or have previously held a consultant position in an NHS hospital.

In the USA they will be or will have been on the medical or surgical staff of a hospital or surgical centre, be allowed to operate and have operating privileges under their speciality. Many will ideally also be on the faculty of one of the medical schools, e.g. I am Clinical Professor of Dermatology at UCLA School of Medicine. A plastic surgeon would be Clinical Professor of Plastic Surgery at a School of Medicine. A Clinical Assistant Professor or Clinical Associate Professor will be less senior or less academically recognised by their medical school than a Professor.

Non-physician cosmetic care

Aestheticians and beauty therapists

These should be certified by training boards. Some may be trained in private institutions and others at colleges. They should have a diploma from Cidesco (*Comité Internationale d'Esthétique et de cosmétologie*) and/or BABTAC (British Association of Beauty Therapy and Cosmetology) and/or City and Guilds, requiring a training period of between three months and three years. Officially they are permitted to do facial and body treatments, including some microdermabrasion, milder peels, acne extraction, electrolysis, manicures, hair removal (using electrolysis and pulsed light), as well as offer advice on sun protection and non-prescription skin products. They are not legally allowed to give injections or provide prescription medication. Because there are different levels of training, however, it is important to check carefully before embarking on any course of treatment.

Sadly, and potentially dangerously, some therapists advise on dermatology treatments and perform procedures that can result in side effects that they are not equipped to solve. On the other hand, well-trained aestheticians and beauty therapists working with dermatologists can be very helpful, especially in advising and instructing the patients in sun protection and cream application and in answering some questions. They do not however attempt to diagnose moles or give opinions on skin conditions.

---

* Appropriate questions to ask when choosing a practitioner *

- *Do they have malpractice medical insurance coverage?* This may seem an unnecessary question but, in fact, many practitioners and nurses are not covered by medical insurance companies for practising cosmetic procedures, and should anything go wrong you will have some difficulty gaining recompense.

- *Do they have specialist training in relevant areas of medicine and surgery?* Have them show you certificates and take the time to check these and other credentials thoroughly. In the UK check with the GMC. In the USA check with the speciality academy (see pages 151–152).

- *Do I really need, or will I really benefit from, the procedure(s) in question?* Ask to be put in touch with and to see photographs of patients they have treated.

Cosmetic specialists

This title can refer to anything from a beauty therapist to someone who has worked in a dermatology or plastic surgeon's clinic and feels they have seen and learned enough to qualify them to offer advice to patients. Some work by referring to physicians and surgeons, who may be expected to give a percentage of their fee in return. This is illegal in the USA, but surprisingly can happen in the UK.

Cosmetic surgeon, cosmetic physician

May mean anything from a General Practitioner, internist to even a pathologist who has decided cosmetic surgery is more rewarding or lucrative than their original practice and have 're-branded' themselves. No specific proof of training or expertise is required.

Nurses – dermatology and cosmetic

Dermatology-trained nurses first gain a general nursing degree and experience, then train in assisting dermatologists in the treatment of skin diseases and in performing cosmetic and surgery procedures. They make an invaluable contribution to the smooth functioning of a clinic, not least in preparing patients for procedures by answering certain questions and helping to put them at ease. However, a bizarre loophole in the system in the UK means that some nurses are allowed to administer injections of fillers and Botox, on the basis that these procedures are 'non-invasive'. Unfortunately, they do not have the necessary training or expertise to deal with complications that may arise and should not, therefore, undertake such procedures.

Cosmetic dentist

A more worrying trend is for dentists to claim they can perform cosmetic procedures on the face, but beware: they often may not have had more than a weekend course of training and in the UK there is a severe shortage of dentists willing to do dentistry!

General practitioner (GP)

In the UK they may take an interest in dermatology. GPs will have trained at medical school as physicians and then undertaken two to three years of GP training. Most have little dermatology training, as unfortunately, dermatology is only taught for two to four weeks at medical schools. A few will have served as Clinical Assistants in dermatology in NHS hospitals and will be experienced – my London associate Dr Anne Maxwell was a GP but also spent 14 years as a Clinical Assistant in dermatology at a university hospital.

There is no equivalent in the USA as you have to be fully trained and certified in dermatology (see above) to claim specialist expertise.

Important associations and contacts for information about cosmetic procedures and physicians

In the UK

British Association of Dermatologists
19 Fitzroy Square, London W1T 6EH
020 7383 0266
admin@bad.org.uk
www.bad.org.uk

British Society for Dermatological Surgery
As above

British Association of Plastic Surgeons
The Royal College of Surgeons
35–43 Lincoln's Inn Fields, London
WC2A 3PN
020 7831 5161/2
secretariat@baps.co.uk
www.baps.co.uk

British Association of Aesthetic Plastic Surgeons
The Royal College of Surgeons of England
35–43 Lincoln's Inn Fields, London
WC2A 3PN
020 7405 2234

General Medical Council
178 Great Portland Street, London W1W 5JE
020 7580 7642
gmc@gmc-uk.org
www.gmc-uk.org

Royal College of Physicians
11 St Andrews Place, Regent's Park,
London NW1 4LE
020 7935 1174

Royal College of Surgeons of England
35–43 Lincoln's Inn Fields, London
WC2A 3PE
020 7405 3474

Royal College of Surgeons in Edinburgh
Nicholson Street, Edinburgh EH8 9DW
0131 527 1600
mail@rcsed.ac.uk
information@rcsed.ac.uk
www.rcsed.ac.uk

Royal College of Surgeons in Ireland
123 St Stephens Green, Dublin 2, Ireland
353 1 402 2100
info@rcsi.ie
www.rcsi.ie

In Europe

European Academy of Dermatology (EADV)
A Fellow of the EADV has been fully trained and recognised as a specialist dermatologist from one of the European medical schools – equivalent to American and British dermatologists.

Ave Général de Gaulle 38, B1050 Brussels, Belgium

+32 2 650 00 98

In the USA

American Board of Dermatology
Henry Ford Health System
1 Ford Place, Detroit, Michigan 48202-3450
313-874-1088
abderm@hfhs.org
www.abderm.org

American Academy of Dermatology
PO Box 4014, Schaumburg
IL 60168-4014
847-330-0230
www.aad.org

American Society for Dermatologic Surgery
5550 Meadowbrook Drive, Suite 120
Rolling Meadows, IL 60008
847-956-0900
info@asds.net
www.asds-net.org

American Board of Plastic Surgery
Seven Penn Center, Suite 400
1635 Market Street, Philadelphia, PA 19103-2204
215-587-9322
info@abplsurg.org   www.abplsurg.org

American Academy of Cosmetic Surgery
Cosmetic Surgery Information Service
737 N. Michigan Ave, Suite 820, Chicago, IL 60611
312-981-6760
info@cosmeticsurgery.org
www.cosmeticsurgery.org

American Academy of Facial Plastic and Reconstructive Surgery
310 S. Henry Street, Alexandria, VA 22314
703 299-9291
(800) 332-FACE
info@aafprs.org
www.facial-plastic-surgery.org

American Board of Ophthalmology
111 Presidential Boulevard, Suite 241
Bala Cynwyd, PA 19004–1075
610-664-1175
info@abop.org
www.abop.org

American Academy of Otolaryngology
One Prince Street
Alexandria,
VA 22314
703-836-4444
www.entnet.org

Other associations a physician or surgeon may be listed under

American Society of Lasers in Medicine and Surgery (ASLMS)

European Society of Laser Aesthetic Surgery (ESLD)

European Society of Laser Dermatology (ESLAS)

International Society of Cosmetic Laser Surgeons (ISCLS)

Trained electrolygists should belong to the American Electrology Association

These organisations will tell you something about the skills and training of the physician or surgeon, but only if you first understand the guidelines of these societies. For example, I am a *Fellow* of the American Academy of Cosmetic Surgery (FAACS) which means that I was tested by my peers and had to have 100 cosmetic treatments evaluated by the Academy for satisfactory performance. However, any physician can become a *member* of the American Academy of Cosmetic Surgery without undergoing an evaluation of their expertise. The same applies to the various laser societies (non-physicians and surgeons can become members of some of these but not full fellows).

Yet other associations have been set up without review by the specialist authorities. For example, the British Cosmetic Physician Association has doctors who may be interested in the cosmetic treatments, but who will not have undergone approved, supervised specialist training. It is not recognised by the General Medical Council.

glossary of skin-care terms

Acid mantle

This refers to the fact that the surface of the skin is slightly acidic, i.e. it has a mantle or coating of acidity (the pH of the skin is 5.5).

AHAs

Alpha-hydroxy acids (fruit acids) are derived from fruit and milk sugars and are often added to skin-care products. They can improve oily skin, treat fine lines and wrinkles and improve skin texture.

Collagen

Collagen is the largest part of the skin's support structure and, in particular, in the *dermis* (see chapter 1). It is closely associated with the elastic fibres and it gives the skin its resilience, normal stretching and strength.

Cortisone

This is a type of hormone or steroid-like medicine that has very excellent and profound anti-inflammatory properties. It is a very frequent ingredient in many of the creams that are used in inflamed skin conditions such as eczema or psoriasis, but some of the mid-strength and stronger cortisone creams can thin the skin if used for long periods of time.

Cosmeceuticals

This is a term that was coined about 15 years ago and denotes a product, e.g. glycolic acid, that is at a strength where it is not considered a pharmaceutical product and therefore is not regulated as a medicine but is thought or known to have a definite benefit or effect on the skin. You can obtain cosmeceuticals without a prescription.

Dermatitis

Any inflamed red skin condition, including common types such as eczema or psoriasis.

Dermis

This is the underlay below the *epidermis*.

The dermis contains *collagen* and *elastin* and is important in feeding and supplying the nerve endings for the skin. It is the support structure for the epidermis.

Elastin

This is the second-most important substance in the *dermis* after *collagen*. Its normal function, when undamaged, is to give the skin elasticity and resilience and to prevent skin looseness. Elastin is frequently damaged by repeated exposure to sunlight, particularly long-wave *ultraviolet* A, and also by inflammation, e.g. acne.

Electrolytes

The chemicals that make up the contents of the body; the common electrolytes are sodium, potassium and chloride. It is important that these are present in correct amounts for the body to function.

Epidermis

This is the outer layer of the skin which protects the skin and contains the skin barrier, the *stratum corneum*.

Eumelanin

The commonest form of *melanin*, present in all human skin except for redheads. It is produced by the pigment cells or *melanocytes* and is important for the production of skin pigment as well as protection from sun exposure. It also has an antioxidant to mop up *free radicals*.

Fibroblast

These are cells that are found in the *dermis* and are very important as the main producers of *collagen* and *elastin*. They can be stimulated in various ways, for example with creams containing Retin-A or with certain lasers to produce more collagen and therefore skin rejuvenation.

Free radicals

These are damaging chemicals that are released by exposure to *ultraviolet* or to chemicals. Free radicals damage a variety of skin functions, leading to cell damage, premature ageing and possibly increased risk of cancer.

Humectant

A moisture-attracting ingredient, e.g. glycerine.

Hypertrophic

A thickening or increased size of a skin or other lesion. One example is a thickened red hypertrophic scar, very common in certain parts of the skin, for example on the front of the chest after heart surgery.

Keloid scars

A raised red scar that is thicker and spreads more widely than a hypertrophic scar. Both hypertrophic and keloid scars are thought to be a result of too much *fibroblast* activity producing thickened *collagen*.

Keratinocyte

The main cell of the *epidermis* which produces the protective layer or barrier of the skin, the *stratum corneum*. There are 10 keratinocytes to every 1 pigment-forming cell or *melanocyte*. The *melanin* that is produced by the melanocyte is transferred into the keratinocytes for optimum protection in response to sunlight.

Mask of pregnancy

These are dark patches on the face, in

particular, the cheeks, nose, upper lip and forehead that can occur in women after pregnancy or from taking the contraceptive pill or hormone replacement therapy.

Melanin

The substance the skin produces to give a tan. This has important pigmentation and protective qualities that also give an antioxidant ability which reduces *free radical* production. Melanin is produced most efficiently in black skin.

Melanocytes

This is the pigment-producing factory of the skin, responsible for producing *melanin*.

Melanoma

A potentially lethal but also curable cancer if detected early, arising from the *melanocyte* pigment cells in the skin.

Nasolabial folds

These are the folds that run between the outside angles of the mouth and the nose.

Phaeomelanin

This is the type of *melanin* that is present in red-headed people. This is a much less efficient type of melanin, as it does not produce a tan of any protectiveness or colour. Nor is it as efficient at quenching *free radicals* – see *eumelanin*.

Photoageing

This is the process by which the skin undergoes accelerated ageing after *ultraviolet* exposure.

Precancerous skin spots (solar keratoses)

These are red, scaling rough patches, some of which may also be pigmented, that appear on sun-exposed skin (the back of the hands, the face and the forehead). It is important that these are examined and treated because 14 per cent go on to become squamous cell cancer.

Retinoid

One of a group of pharmaceutical substances related to vitamin A and known as retinoids or vitamin-A derivatives. They have very important rejuvenation effects on the skin.

Sebaceous gland

The oil-producing glands that are attached to the hair follicles, most common on the face and upper body.

Stratum corneum

This is the outermost layer of the *epidermis* and protects the skin from external toxins as well as reducing the loss of water and *electrolytes* from within.

Subcutaneous tissue

This is the supporting structure under the dermis that contains fat, blood vessels, muscles and nerves. It is a vital part of the normal contour of the skin and body. When subcutaneous tissue is lost, i.e. with loss of fat, this can accelerate the ageing process and it has also been implicated in problems on the body, such as cellulite.

Sunspots (lentigo)

Flat, brown spots, regular in colour and usually benign (i.e. non-cancerous).

Seborrhoeic keratoses

These are often unsightly, crusted and braced, sometimes with brown or pigmented lumps or white, scaly, raised patches. They are benign but can be confusing to non-dermatologists as they can mimic *melanoma* and other skin cancer.

Trichology

This is the science of studying hair growth and diseases of the hair. Dermatologists are trained in all diseases of the skin, hair and nails. Trichologists are non-physicians who have taken a diploma or course about the hair and scalp.

Ultraviolet

Ultraviolet radiation is the part of the sun's spectrum that is between the x-rays and the visible spectrum. The lowest wavelength of the visible spectrum is violet in colour, hence the term ultraviolet.

acknowledgements

I am very grateful for the advice and suggestions of Muna Reyal and Anne Newman and to Kyle Cathie, the publisher. They have all been so encouraging, patient and helpful with the production and editing of this book.

I am forever indebted to my understanding and uniquely talented wife, Pamela, for organising my busy life between our clinical centres in London and Santa Monica. Her words of wisdom are always to be noted and ignored at my peril!

I am fortunate to have my two beautiful daughters, Nichola and Philippa, as an inspiration for my life and work. I want to thank Philippa, a physician and now an attorney, for her help, wisdom, research assistance and for having our granddaughter Annie. Little Annie keeps us all very active and youthful – she is a wonderful gift for us all.

I would like to thank the many patients I have seen in my dermatology practice over the last 30 years who have allowed me to consult, advise and treat them. They have placed their trust in me and I have tried not to disappoint them. I continue to strive to achieve the best possible outcome for my patients and always try to inform them accurately and give the most appropriate treatments. Patient education is, I believe, a keystone for responsible medicine.

Finally, I want to acknowledge that I have consulted for and conducted research with some of the companies that have developed treatments discussed in this book.

I hope my readers will find this book of help in exploring what is a rapidly evolving area of practice, allowing us to offer so much more today than we could just a few years ago.

picture credits

Page 1 Image Source/Alamy; 2 Saturn Stills/Science Photo Library; 6 Image Source/Alamy; 8 Francesca Yorke; 9 Getty Images/Christopher Thomas; 10 Coneyl Jay/Science Photo Library; 12 Robert Updegraff; 13 Andrew Syred/Science Photo Library; 16 Robert Updegraff; 17 BSIP Jolyot/Science Photo Library; 22 Coneyl Jay/Science Photo Library; 24 Coneyl Jay/Science Photo Library; 25 BananaStock/Alamy (top), Coneyl Jay/Science Photo Library (bottom); 26 BananaStock/Alamy (top), Image Source/Alamy (bottom); 27 Bluestone/Science Photo Library; 28 RubberBall/Alamy (top), BananaStock/Alamy (middle), RubberBall/Alamy (bottom); 29 Pixland/Alamy (top), BananaStock/Alamy (middle), BananaStock/Alamy (bottom); 31 Cristina Pedrazzini/Science Photo Library; 32 Lauren Shear/Science Photo Library; 33 Coneyl Jay/Science Photo Library; 34 Lauren Shear/Science Photo Library; 36 Sheila Tarry/Science Photo Library; 38 BSIP, Chassenet/Science Photo Library; 45 Dr Nicholas Lowe; 46 BSIP, Laurent/Science Photo Library; 49 Dr Nicholas Lowe; 56 Dr Nicholas Lowe; 58 Dr Nicholas Lowe; 62 Dr Nicholas Lowe; 68 Zefa; 73 Dr Nicholas Lowe; 74 Dr Nicholas Lowe; 81 BSIP, Laurent/Louise Eve/Science Photo Library; 86 Dr Nicholas Lowe; 94 Zefa; 96 William Lingwood/Science Photo Library; 97 Vaseline Intensive Care Essential Moisture Lotion; 99 TH Foto-Werbung/Science Photo Library; 100 BSIP, Chassenet/Science Photo Library; 102 Erich Schrempp/Science Photo Library; 104 Michelle Garrett; 110 Getty Images/Ron Chapple; 111 David Raymer/Corbis; 115 Image Source/Alamy; 116 Cristina Pedrazzini/Science Photo Library; 118 Dr P. Marazzi/Science Photo Library; 119 Gordon Garradd/Science Photo Library; 120 Untitled/Alamy; 121 PhotoDisc; 122 Geoff Hayes; 123 PhotoDisc; 124 BananaStock/Alamy; 126 David Munns/Science Photo Library; 128 Bonnie Sue Rauch/Science Photo Library; 129 John Cole/Science Photo Library; 130 Goodshoot/Alamy; 133 Image Source/Alamy; 136 S.T. Yiap/Alamy; 137 BSIP Collet/Science Photo Library; 138 H. Raguet/Eurelios/Science Photo Library; 140 H. Raguet/Eurelios/Science Photo Library; 141 L'Oréal/Eurelios/Science Photo Library; 143 Robert Leon/Alamy

index